Some Early Reactions

- "I am certain the book will be well received and will be a valuable source of information for people in the healing process....I hope it reaches a very wide audience." - Bob Soderlund, Editor, *Ha-Shilth-Sa*, Nuu-chah-nulth newspaper, Port Alberni, B.C.

- "There are no them and us; there is only us. The book reminds me of that. These are my brothers and sisters." - Don Vipond, Editorial-Page Editor, *Times-Colonist*, Victoria, B.C.

- "As I read...my heart grew warmer and warmer as I relived the rough beginning and the gradual growth and development of Ka Ka Wis." - Lorraine LaMarre, SSA, Lachine, Quebec.

- "***Healing Journeys***....provides a working model for rehabilitation programs with its emphasis upon the natives themselves, their self-help resources and objectives within the family circle." - James Gray, OSB, St. Peter's Abbey, Muenster, Sask.

- "The story is essentially that of a God-given, life-changing idea....It makes stirring reading all the way." Frederick (Ted) B. Watt, author, Victoria.

- "Much of the strength...of ***Healing Journeys*** is in its openness to drawing both from traditional (aboriginal) spirituality and Christianity....I think we all have a long way to go in our understanding of how the Great Spirit/Holy Spirit is at work." - Peter Flemington, Program Director VISION/TV, Toronto.

- "Congratulations on ***Healing Journeys***.... I expect it will be a success from every point of view." - Vince La Plante, OMI, Vancouver.

- "I am drawn by compassion into the story. I note the need of the people and their pain. I appreciate the numerous anecdotes which help me know the people and relate to them....Each of the success stories is a beacon." - Arden Wells Moretti, free-lance writer, Victoria.

- "I think the telling of this story important. Of such efforts are myths made. The white myths too long have devalued native people's lives." - Dr. John Thompson, President, St. Thomas More College, University of Saskatchewan, Saskatoon, Sask.

Healing Journeys

The Ka Ka Wis Experience 1974 – 1994

dear Gerry:
I await your verdict
with much interest.
Granton

**Published by the Ka Ka Wis Family Development Centre
as part of our 20th Anniversary celebrations
and renewed commitment to widen the Circle of Healing.**

1994

Canadian Cataloguing in Publication Data

Main entry under title:

Healing Journeys

ISBN 0-9698217-0-0

1. Ka Ka Wis Family Development Centre--History. 2. Substance abuse--Patients--Rehabilitation--British Columbia--Meares Island. 3. Indians of North America--Drug abuse--British Columbia--Meares Island. 4. Indians of North America--Alcohol use--British Columbia--Meares Island. I. Ka Ka Wis Family Development Centre.

RC564.75.C2H42 1994   616.86'03'097112   C94-910488-4

First printing June 1994.

Healing Journeys is published by the Ka Ka Wis Family Development Centre, Box 17, Tofino, B.C. V0R 2Z0.

Readers are welcome to reproduce and distribute printed material from this book. We would appreciate acknowledgement of this source when so doing. - *The Editorial Team.*

Production, including overall design, cover illustration, colour art reproduction and camera-ready type was provided by:
Express Editorial & Graphics Ltd.,
356 Cyril Owen Place,
R.R. 3
Victoria, B.C. V8X 3X1

Printing was produced by:
Kromar Printing Ltd.,
725 Portage Avenue
Winnipeg, Man. R3G 0M8

ISBN 0 - 9698217 - 0 - 0

Table of Contents

Introduction 1
    Dedication 3
    Foreword 5
    Guest Comments...6
    The Editorial Team, The Artists, Acknowledgements 8
    Why Ka Ka Wis Matters..10
A History in the Making...13
    "Ka Ka Wis" — The Name and the Meaning.................................14
    The Curtain Tells the Story..14
    Some Highlights and Profiles...17
        The First and Only Mayor...17
        A New Vision: The Kyuquot Proposal 19
        Pioneer Hopes and Plans..20
        Life Before and After: Mabel's Story...23
        Top Priorities: Safety and Health 28
        The Night Old Christie Burned 30
        Children Heal Dark Memories..32
        A Celebration of Native Culture 35
        Life and Work on an Island..36
    Problem and Solution..39
    Client Voices I: Speaking from the Heart......................................39
    Memories of the Early Years 41
    Reasons to Celebrate 45
    Poems I: The Laureate of Ka Ka Wis..48
The Evolving Program 51
    Philosophy and Mission...52
    "A Program Like None Other" 53
    The Current Program 54
    Quality Assurance 58
    The Silent Crew 60
    Memories and Reflections on Program..61
    Feelings 64
    Client Voices II..65
    Trainees..67
    Smudgings and Sweats 68
    The Learning Centre 71
    A Postscript 76
    More Reasons to Celebrate...76
    Single Moms' Session 80
    TFN Experiment: Three Views 82

Other Centres 84
"What's Your Success Rate?" 85
Two Other Views of "Success" 87
Poems II: Three by Three 88
Healing — Experienced and Shared 91
Where's Healing? 92
Someone Special 93
"The Circle is Sacred" 93
My Journey So Far: Joe's Story 95
The Blue Bead Ceremony 99
Client Voices III 101
More Recent Memories 103
Island Bridges 107
Concerns, Hopes and Celebrations 109
Will the Bridge Hold? 114
Both Partners Need the Bridge 122
A Fragile Strength 124
Serenity Prayer 125
The Bigger Picture: Where Ka Ka Wis Fits In 127
I Aboriginal Families — The First Pioneers 128
II Christian Missions and Christie School 1874-1971 134
    Three Postscripts to the Christie School Story: 142
    1 Students' and Teachers' Memories 142
    2 Paint the Whole Picture! 146
    3 Towards a Balanced Viewpoint 148
III Ka Ka Wis: Healing Circle for Families 1974-94 149
IV What of the Future? Some Possibilities 177
Names and Numbers 179
Some Names are Missing 180
Why "Clients"? 180
Members, Board of Directors 181
Core Community, Centre Staff and Volunteers 182
Sample Program Exercise 185
The Ka Ka Wis Foundation Fund 186

Introduction

Dedication

Healing Journeys is dedicated to the memories of five persons who fought valiantly against substance addiction before their untimely deaths:

Matilda Leo

Jack Ryan, OMI

Sarah Williams

A Young Married Couple

The unnamed aboriginal couple were among the first to plant the fruitful seed that later became the Ka Ka Wis Family Development Centre. In 1971 the husband shared this young couple's hopeful dream with their pastor. Later the priest recalled the family man's words: "Padre...why don't you do something with Old Christie School now that it's closed? Make a centre out of it for people like my wife and me, so we can go there for treatment and bring the family with us." Tragically, both husband and wife died from alcoholism before the new Centre opened a few years later.

These pages are also dedicated to all family members and individuals who since 1974 have joined the Ka Ka Wis Circle in search of inner healing, and to all who will join this quest in days to come. Before all others, this book is your story.

Introduction 5

Foreword

By Patrick Koreski, Executive Director
   Qʷayac̓iik

I believe Ka Ka Wis is an example of justice in action and co-operation in doing. As a white male who worked at the Christie Residential School, I am glad to have had the opportunity to help right some of the wrongs of the past, while remembering some of the good things that also happened. I am especially glad I can do this with many of the same people from residential school days.

Since the Family Development Centre began in 1974, many "white" staff have worked long hours with little financial gain, and mostly out of their personal commitment to the cause. Without this dedication and commitment, Ka Ka Wis would not be a reality today. This I believe and I am proud to be part of this group.

Not that I or other members of the dominant society have worked harder or can claim more credit for what Ka Ka Wis has become. Not at all. Ka Ka Wis is what it is primarily because of the natives who have worked here and who have come here as clients. The rest of us listened and walked with our aboriginal neighbours to support them and encourage what happened.

Both cultures came together and we have Ka Ka Wis as it is now. Both cultures have reason to be proud of Ka Ka Wis. And especially to be proud of working together. In the final analysis Ka Ka Wis is not just a place or a program but people working with people. **Healing Journeys** is about these people.

Guest Comments

Francis Frank, Chief Councillor, Tla O Qui Aht First Nations

Healing Journeys reveals how the experiences of First Nations' peoples at Ka Ka Wis and how Ka Ka Wis itself have both come full circle. The reflections show how our people have made positive choices and tremendous changes in their own lives, so that each person is walking down a path of hope, strength and happiness.

Gone are the days of constant blaming of others for the way we are as individuals or families. The reflections in this book show that many First Nations peoples have taken their own initiatives to change their futures, instead of just living on how bad their past has been.

Gone also are the days of other people feeling they know what is best for First Nations individuals and families. More representative of what First Nations people are like today are those individuals and families who decided for themselves what is best. Many have chosen Ka Ka Wis as the site to embark on that healing journey.

Gone are images of Ka Ka Wis as a site where families were torn apart. Instead, many now view and envisage the strength, hope and happiness the site holds when families are drawn together. What the site once stood for has been passed over and replaced by the healing journeys many First Nation peoples have chosen to make.

It was in this positive spirit that ***Healing Journeys*** was developed. The book reflects how many people's lives have developed and also how Ka Ka Wis has developed. First Nations peoples and Ka Ka Wis have journeyed together to strengthen families and individuals. There is a shared sense of hope and happiness in knowing that we have taken a new direction towards a new future together.

Introduction

Bishop Remi J. De Roo, Roman Catholic Diocese of Victoria

On February 3, 1962, shortly after my arrival on Vancouver Island, the native tribes honoured me by adopting me as a brother. They gave me the name of High Priest White Swan. That was the beginning of very rewarding contacts with First Nations peoples in this region.

Ka Ka Wis has been at the heart of my growing understanding of the relationships between native spirituality and the biblical faith which is our common Christian heritage.

People familiar with the early history of the Pacific west coast know that pastoral concern for the spiritual well-being of the aboriginal peoples was one of the main preoccupations of Bishop Demers, founder of our Diocese.

Some aspects of the early missionary endeavours, once taken for granted, today are judged as culturally distorted and misguided. We regret the mistakes of the past and seek to make amends for them, just as we mourn the passing of yesterday's world. Let us not tarry there. Attributing guilt for previous failings only imprisons us in our common human problems. We liberate ourselves and others by appropriate mourning, reconciliation and renewed common endeavours on the paths of hope. Ka Ka Wis has much to teach us in this regard. I welcome these moving stories in ***Healing Journeys***. I applaud and thank their authors.

Vatican II celebrated the presence of the Holy Spirit among all peoples yet to be evangelized. Divine grace left its traces in all ancient civilizations, long before the advent of the earliest missionaries. Our native brothers and sisters, whether baptized or not, can enrich us through their heritage even as they receive from and with us the Good News of Christ, incarnate, crucified, risen.

Telling our stories is an excellent way to develop partnerships in exploring the ways of God in our midst. By sharing our dreams we will become more conscious of the ways of divine Providence and marvel at the gracious purpose of our Creator. This is indeed the Lord's work, drawing good even out of evil (*Psalm* 118). Let us embrace one another, join hands and move forward together as "pilgrims of the Absolute".

8   *Healing Journeys*

The Editorial Team

Pat Koreski - I like to think that my claim to fame is that I am Colleen's husband and the father of Jennifer, Kate, Kelly and Jeremy. I immigrated from "the States" in 1970 and have lived in or near Tofino since then. Originally I worked at Christie, and then was a commercial fisherman for 10 years. I have been the director of Ka Ka Wis since the fall of 1982. It has been a challenge, at times damn frustrating, but I feel very honoured and privileged to have been part of the Expanding Circle. I feel our Creator is primarily in charge here. Choo.

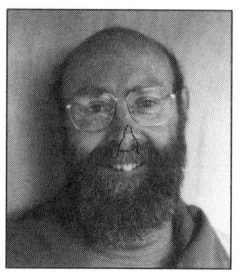

Mabel James - My name is Mabel James and I am an alcoholic. My tribe is the Kwicksutaineuk people. I am the mother of four and the Grandmother of seven. I reached grade ten in school. I attended residential school in Alert Bay. In 1982 my family and I came to Ka Ka Wis for treatment. A year later my husband and I were hired as workers here, him in maintenance and me in the Daycare and later as a counsellor. Between the lines there has been much pain, as well as many things conquered. I love life and it loves me. I love to share my life with whoever will listen. It is my way of saying, "There is hope."

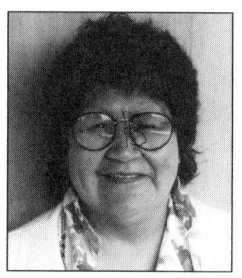

George Atleo - I was born and raised in Ahousat, B.C. until I attended Port Alberni Residential School from 1964 to 1968. I boarded and then lived with my mother in my last year at school. I graduated in 1970. Was employed as a mill worker, 1971-83. Then I accepted a challenging position as Executive Director of the Port Alberni Friendship Centre from 1983 to 1987. I moved back to the west coast, and was employed as a fish-plant worker until 1990. That year I was employed at Ka Ka Wis as a maintenance worker. Since 1991, with an interest in and commitment to all aspects of the program, I have worked as a personal and family addictions counsellor. I have four children from a previous marriage: Margaret, Georgette, Carol-Ann and George Jr. My lovely wife

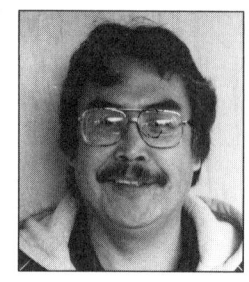

Marie and I have two children: Nellie and Randall. For us, Ka Ka Wis has given us a new discovery in "Life".

Grant Maxwell - After 40-plus years as a reporter, researcher and editor in three provinces, this Saskatchewan-born family man and my wife Vivian retired to Vancouver Island in 1987. Very soon the "retiree" was busy on new assignments. Since October, 1992, for example, I have worked many hundreds of hours as editor and main writer of *Healing Journeys*. Why? What "hooked me"? Well, first of all, the chance to spread the 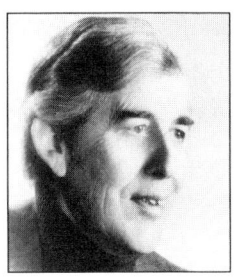 good news about Ka Ka Wis at a time when headlines and newscasts are playing up the bad news day after day. Second, I expected to enjoy working with the Centre team and hoped to learn much by interviewing dozens of men and women belonging to two cultures. This proved true on both counts. The extra income was helpful. And this 71-year-old could not resist the creative challenge. I felt called by the Spirit to say "Yes," and I'm thankful I did.

The Artists

Several gifted persons are responsible for the visual content and general presentation of this book. Aboriginal artist **Cecil Dawson** created several of the black and white drawings, as did **Maureen Cato**, Ladysmith. **Bob Cato**, her husband, prepared the detailed map. The photographic overview of the Ka Ka Wis site was taken by **Kevin Timney,** Tofino. **Mark Hobson**, Tofino, photographed the Centre's Dance Curtain. The cover and overall design of the book was created by **Don Lindenberg** of Express Editorial & Graphics, Victoria.

Acknowledgements

Generous assistance by many generous persons in assessing early drafts, reading proofs and helping in other ways to prepare *Healing Journeys* for publication is gratefully acknowledged. There is not enough space to name all who gave a helping hand. Two merit particular thanks: Margaret Cantwell, SSA, and Frank Moretti.

Why Ka Ka Wis Matters

By Grant Maxwell, Editor

From 1900 until 1971 several generations of aboriginal children on Vancouver Island's west coast attended Christie Residential School on Meares Island. Today the same beautiful setting near Tofino is the site of the Ka Ka Wis Family Development Centre. During two decades of struggle and growth this "Circle of Healing" has helped hundreds of native families mend lives previously disrupted by alcoholism, drug addiction, domestic violence, and sometimes by earlier school experiences.

Louie Frank of Ahousat, once a pupil at Christie, now a respected elder and grandfather, speaks joyfully of the difference Ka Ka Wis has made in the lives of many neighbours and relatives. In his words: "Walking around there, my mind flashed back to my residential school days. It was okay....but I was homesick, there's no two ways about it.

"What a contrast between me and my grandchildren! They'll probably think of Ka Ka Wis as the place where they first started being a real family, after my daughter and her husband went there and got turned around....In my case, it was the place where I had to be away from my parents. I'm so grateful my grandchildren can always go back there and say, 'This is where our family came together'. I can't help feeling good about it. I just say a prayer of thanks every chance I get."

Three generations of this family's history sum up the Christie-to-Ka Ka Wis transition! And Louie Frank, an abstainer himself, is by no means alone in feeling thankful. Hear a native grandmother: "My grandchildren are the first generation in our family to live in a drug- and alcohol-free environment. I thank the Creator and you wonderful workers at Ka Ka Wis for that."

Good news like this gets around. So a teen-ager came to Ka Ka Wis with this expectation: " Me and my cousins are on drugs and into stealing and on probation and stuff. I want to make it stop." A younger boy wrote: "My Mom really wants to quit drugs so me and my brother can live a better life. That's why we came to Ka Ka Wis."

Introduction **11**

And a young woman speaks for hundreds of client couples who face their inner pain and deal with it at Ka Ka Wis: "Thanks to our circle for letting me learn how to deal with my anger deep in my heart about men. I know it was from an experience in my early childhood. I accept that now. I am not blaming my parents anymore. I forgave them. The old man also I forgive, and myself. Thanks."

These aboriginal voices and others like them best tell the hope-inspiring story of Ka Ka Wis. They testify to the healing that wounded people experience when they share their pain, pool their strengths and together rely on the Higher Power to see them through.

True, not all or even a majority of clients succeed in overcoming their addiction. Nor is the program fault-free. Despite these human shortcomings, much more has been accomplished at Ka Ka Wis than ever seemed possible when the first clients came to the Centre in 1974.

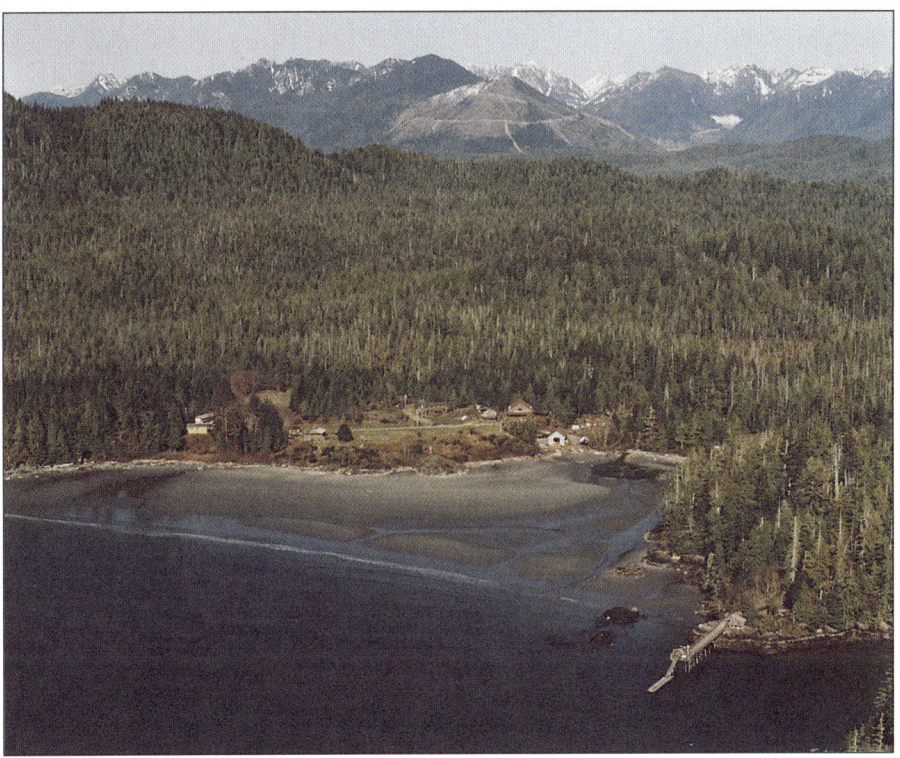

Ka KaWis Family Development Centre

Photo by Kevin Timney

Healing Journeys celebrates these "20 years of transformation" in 1994, which is also the United Nations International Year of the Family. The book anticipates there will be further reasons to celebrate as new goals are reached in future years.

Healing Journeys aspires to spread the good news of the Family Development Centre well beyond Vancouver Island. Why? Because the Ka Ka Wis experience demonstrates one time-tested approach to personal healing, family renewal, and intercultural collaboration. The lessons learned from 20 years of trial-and-error service at Ka Ka Wis have potential significance wherever similar programs are being designed or considered. The Ka Ka Wis experience offers encouragement to every family everywhere that is beleaguered by the demons of addiction.

The Ka Ka Wis story has a Christian component, most noticeably in the Centre's early years. Later an interfaith element came to the fore. Nowadays many Ka Ka Wis participants discover that native spirituality and Christian faith each has inner riches to share with the other, to the benefit of all.

Indeed, this interfaith collaboration reveals that Gospel values and aboriginal ideals have much in common.

A personal note: Because Ka Ka Wis is a beckoning light in a dark and troubled time for many families, I accepted the Centre's invitation to serve as editor of ***Healing Journeys***. It's been hard, and sometimes frustrating work. Even more, it's been a profound learning experience, a life-enhancing endeavor for this "retired" journalist. I am grateful. I hope something of what I experienced first hand will speak deeply to you as you read these pages.

A History in the Making

"Ka Ka Wis" — The Name and the Meaning

"Kakawis" is the usual English spelling of an aboriginal expression that means "place of berries". Why was this name given long ago to the present-day site of the Family Development Centre on Meares Island? Probably because many years ago wild berries grew plentifully along the shoreline and in the nearby woods, just as they do today. Some also think the neighbouring rocky mound on which a large crucifix stands resembles a berry basket — upside down.

In *Healing Journeys* we have changed the usual manner of spelling this place name in an attempt to reflect more accurately the Nuu-chah-nulth pronunciation of the word. A respected coastal elder and cultural teacher, Carrie Little, uses the phonetic spelling of QAA QAA WIS to encourage this pronunciation. We believe "Ka Ka Wis" invites this pronunciation, while retaining the familiar spelling of the place name.

The Curtain Tells The Story

Take a long, thoughtful look at the native work of art opposite. It is known as "The Dance Curtain".

Traditionally, dance curtains depicted the tribal histories of First Nations peoples living on Vancouver Island's west coast. Each curtain belonged to the family of the local chief. This particular curtain belongs to all client families who come to Ka Ka Wis in search of sobriety and peaceful family life. It was presented to the Centre in 1988 by several families, most of them from the region, in appreciation for the healing they had experienced. A tribal dance of celebration in front of the curtain climaxed their traditional presentation of the curtain to Ka Ka Wis.

The 10 by 8 ft. canvas portrays the healing process that happens at the Centre. The red, blue, black and white curtain is the collective work of eight men who created it during spare time while with their families for a counselling session in March-April 1988. The symbolic images, which largely reflect the Nuu-chah-nulth artistic style, speak more eloquently than words. But words help.

Observe and read what the dance curtain portrays, as described by Pat Koreski on the Ka Ka Wis video:

"This dance curtain really does tell our story. On the left we see eight canoes coming to Ka Ka Wis, each bringing a family. We have eight living units here and eight families come at a time for several weeks. Eight families with lots of troubles. They come in small canoes. They come scared of the water. They come scared of the storm. They are in a box, just like the man in the box at bottom left. There are lots of tears, lots of shame, and hanging on to the bottle to try to escape it all.

"But the good thing about this story is not the shame or the fear or the troubled water. What's good is the big canoe. It shows all eight families — men, women and children together in the big canoe. The troubles stay the same, the pain is still there, but now the families can deal with their troubles, with their pain, because they are together in the big safe canoe. If we ride in the canoe long enough, when we get out on the other shore we can take our

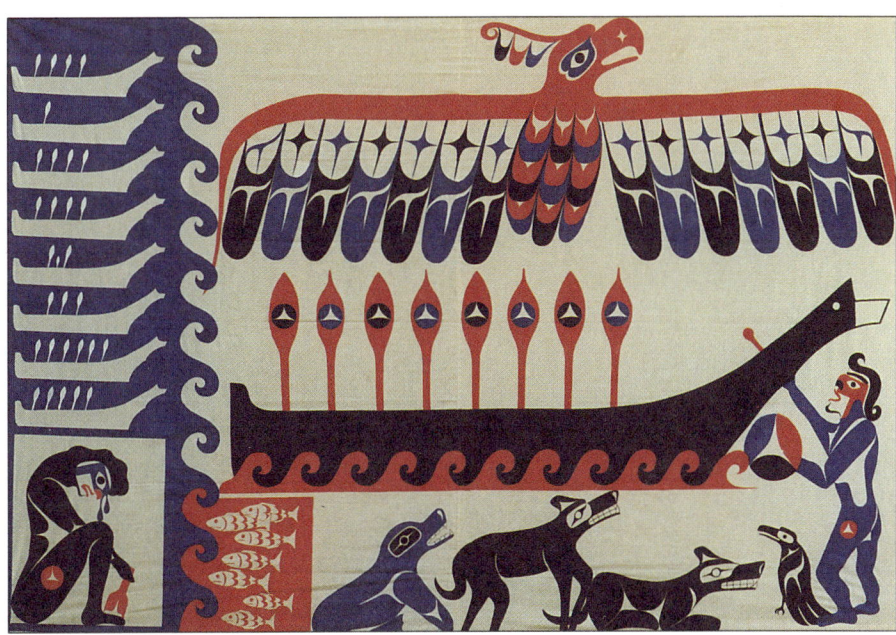

drum and stand up straight as the man is doing, bottom right. We can stand up straight, look up, grab the drum and sing our song.

"I believe we all have songs in our souls, in our very beings, and we need to sing them. If we stay in a box we'll never sing our songs and the world is going to be the worse for it.

"Another beautiful thing about this dance curtain is the Higher Power. I truly believe that at Ka Ka Wis the Higher Power is our centre, gives us energy, gives us life. The Higher Power gives us our song and our Higher Power is there wanting us to sing our song. In the dance curtain the Higher Power is represented by the Thunderbird. Nobody has seen the Thunderbird. Nobody has seen the Higher Power. We carry them in our hearts.

"The dance curtain is a beautiful thing and has lots of energy. It was given to us by clients to remember all the previous clients and to welcome all the future clients. The curtain belongs to Ka Ka Wis; it belongs to all the clients. It's our story."

Kathy Sawyer, later secretary-receptionist at the Centre, added this postscript in the December 1992 issue of the newsletter, the *Ka Ka Wis Star*:

"It was the herring season when the curtain was created. The herrings are shown swimming towards the man in the box to show that herring fishing brings MONEY, ANGER, DANGER, DRINKING....The seal was shot during the herring season and had washed up on the beach. That is why the wolves are on the curtain. They were feeding off the seal. The raven. bottom right, followed the artist around Ka Ka Wis until it also was put on the dance curtain."

Usually at the beginning of each session since its presentation in 1988, the curtain is explained to new client families. It is displayed again for the Blue Bead Ceremony, one of the more stirring events of the Ka Ka Wis program.

The imagery of the dance curtain vividly portrays what this Family Development Centre is about. It both shows and tells the Ka Ka Wis story.

Some Highlights and Profiles

The first chapter of this coastal saga began thousands of years ago with the arrival of the first aboriginal pioneers on Vancouver Island's Pacific shores. Many centuries later, Catholic and Protestant missionaries came. In 1900 Christie Residential School opened on Meares Island. "Old Christie", as it came to be known, closed in 1971. Three years later, the Ka Ka Wis Family Development Centre for native clients opened in the former school buildings.

While ***Healing Journeys*** focuses on the story of the Centre, these pages do not overlook the earlier periods of this ongoing history. A later section, *The Bigger Picture: Where Ka Ka Wis Fits In*, gives an overview of the whole story, including a year-by-year account of the Centre's first two decades. By way of preview, here are some highlights and profiles that give "the feel and flavour" of the Ka Ka Wis story thus far.

The First and Only Mayor

By P.K.

Reg O'Brien — veteran Oblate brother, our unofficial mayor, and a remarkable human being — is definitely one of the reasons to celebrate. Reg has been on site or connected with Ka Ka Wis since 1951. Even those who have mainly negative memories of Christie as a residential school remember Reg as a shining light in a dark experience.

Reg has played a number of tricks or pranks on people during his 40 some years here, and yet lives to tell about it. Reg, although very friendly and outgoing to individuals, is shy of crowds. Perhaps this is because he is a people person and very self-effacing. He neither wants nor strives for crowd approval. He likes people and getting to know people. Reg has the best aptitude or natural ability to counsel of anyone I know. He can pick up strangers hitch-hiking to Port Alberni and have them talking to him about the most intimate details of their lives in five minutes. Why? Because he is sincerely interested in them and their well-being. Reg is a living example of what Ka Ka Wis strives to accomplish.

If a person's wealth is measured by his friends or those who want to be his friend, then Reg is the wealthiest man I know. I am proud to say he was the best man at my wedding, even if he refused to dance at it and broke his promise to me. Reg, thanks for being you, you scoundrel.

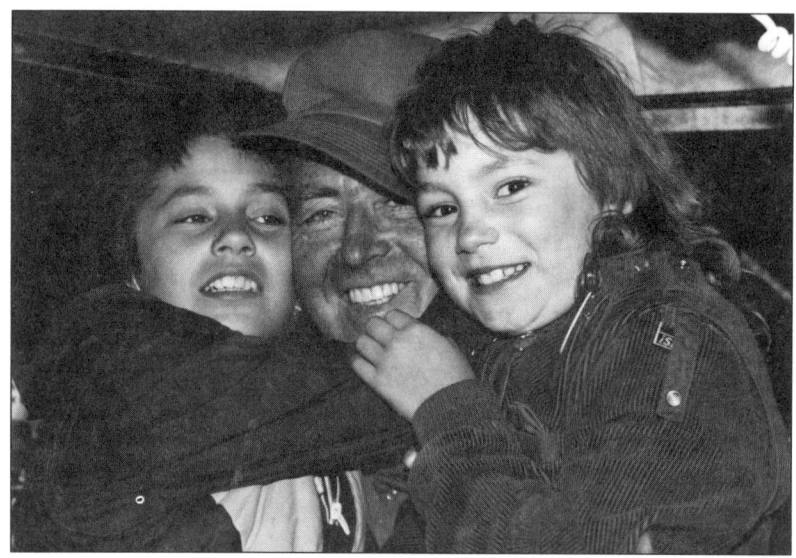

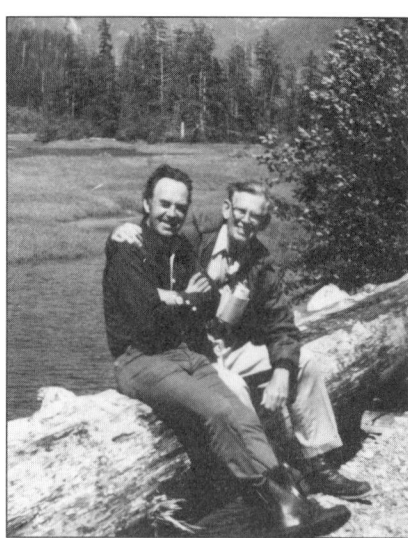

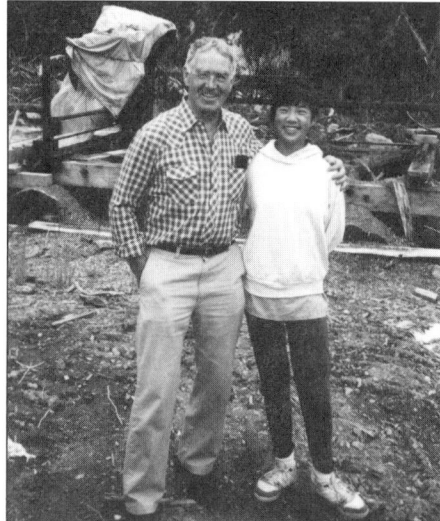

A New Vision: The Kyuquot Proposal

In the fall of 1973 leaders of the Kyuquot tribal band, assisted by pioneer staff living at the Old Christie site, sent a detailed proposal to the B.C. Department of Human Resources. They asked for public funds to operate a new counselling centre, which in hope they had already christened the "Ka Ka Wis Family and Community Development Project".

Here are quotations from the proposal, plus a summary of some findings reported in the submission:

"**Objective**: To provide complete family counselling in an assimilated Indian community. Counselling will cover every aspect of family life — marriage and child counselling and youth counselling, alcohol and drug counselling, health counselling, budgeting and economic counselling. Educational training and counselling will be available to a limited degree as it can be fitted in with the practical operational aspects of the community. Examples of this will be maintenance of boat motors and diesel motors, plumbing, carpentry, possible skiff building, and cooking, gardening, first aid, etc....

"There are more than three families that have expressed the wish to be part of this project by coming to live at Ka Ka Wis and helping out in whatever capacity they can. At present there is one family living there willing to help the project get underway. Also five other people are living there with the same intention.... There have even been several requests by old-age couples to come and help teach and introduce the ways and customs of Indian culture."

The proposal then "documented the needs" found in one west coast community. Of 42 families, 13 were said to have "severe alcoholic problems", 14 had "serious problems" and four "a developing problem". Seven families had "a drug problem". "Serious family breakdown" afflicted 20 households and another four families were tending towards breakdown, the report said.

Nine children had been "apprehended" — taken into custody by social agencies in the past four years. There was evidence of "child neglect" and "possible child battering" in five cases.

Twenty-nine heads of households were employed, but the earning power of 17 of them was "seriously affected by the alcoholic problem". Thirteen family heads were unemployed, 11 of whom "would be employable if they didn't have an alcoholic or family breakdown problem".

Five infant deaths had occurred in the previous two years. Ten children were described as "disturbed". A dozen teenagers were "developing serious problems mainly with alcohol and drugs.

"The above survey presents a very bleak picture of this band," the report said in summing up. "This picture can be duplicated in community after community. Where this Band is exceptional to most bands is that much work has gone into efforts to attack and deal with these problems by the band members themselves."

The report went on to say that the band now employed a welfare aid worker, a community-family life worker and a band homemaker who worked in the homes as needed.

Pioneer Hopes and Plans

Twenty-three trail blazers took part in a two-day winter meeting late in January, 1975 — 17 mostly native supporters and a half dozen members of the fledgling Ka Ka Wis staff. Several months after the first clients had come to the new Centre, members of "the core community and support group" met to exchange information and ideas, hopes and concerns.

Responses to three basic questions were reported in the *Minutes* prepared by Sister Lorraine LaMarre, SSA. Here is a record of pioneer expectations when the Family Development Centre was beginning its second year of service. Excerpts from Lorraine's report:

- "What do you think of this project? — Amazement and congratulations expressed at the progress made in short time. Strength seen in Whites and Indians working together. We Indians should not be hung up on 'taking over'.... Appreciation of the concept of spirituality, of closeness to God....
- "What do you think can be done to respond to the needs of people? — Appreciate the deep religious feelings shown by ancestors before Christianity

came and in accepting it. Our people have will power and can use it for self-discipline.... Chiefs must see alcoholism as a sickness and take more responsibility in having it treated.... Maintain contact with villages. Make known Ka Ka Wis is available.

- "Are **you** willing and available to be involved in this project? How? — I will write to chiefs and the (West Coast Native) Council to look into part of the financing. Building is here, equipment is here and willing people.... I will spread information about what is happening at Ka Ka Wis to engender some soul-searching and positive enthusiastic support.... Someone should write a report about Ka Ka Wis for *Ha-Shilth-Sa* (Native Council's newspaper).... I will come some day soon to live here with my family to get help with my problems and then be able to help my fellow man...There will have to be a chartered non-profit organization to handle funds received, if and when monies come."

The 1975 event on January 28-29 began with "a community supper in the big kitchen at Old Christie. After the meal and a social evening of games the first session began at 9.30 PM" with 19 people present. Four more joined the group the next morning. The roll call of visitors in the order listed: Joe and Regina Tom, Barney and Rose Williams, Louie and Eva Frank, Ray Williams, Matthew Williams, Lillian Howard, Irene Wilson, Ray and Sarah Williams, Archie Little, John Lucas, Ruth Little, Mary Hayes, Barney Williams Sr., and Patrick Koreski. Plus the host team of three Oblates of Mary Immaculate (OMI): Fathers Jim MacDonell and Gerry Guillet, plus Brother Tom Cavanaugh; and three Sisters of St. Ann: Mary McGarrigle, Kathy Erickson and Lorraine LaMarre. Because of illness Rev. Lloyd Hooper of the United Church and Sr. Marjorie Kuntz, CSJ, could not attend.

Gerry Guillet opened the evening session. After prayer and words of welcome, Ray and Sarah Williams, Archie Little and John Lucas were heard. "Each spoke of the problem areas recognized in his or her life, of the help received at Ka Ka Wis, of the family feeling here, of the return to God and the practice of faith, and of the desire to help others regain peace of mind. They felt they were taking part in the making of history at Ka Ka Wis."

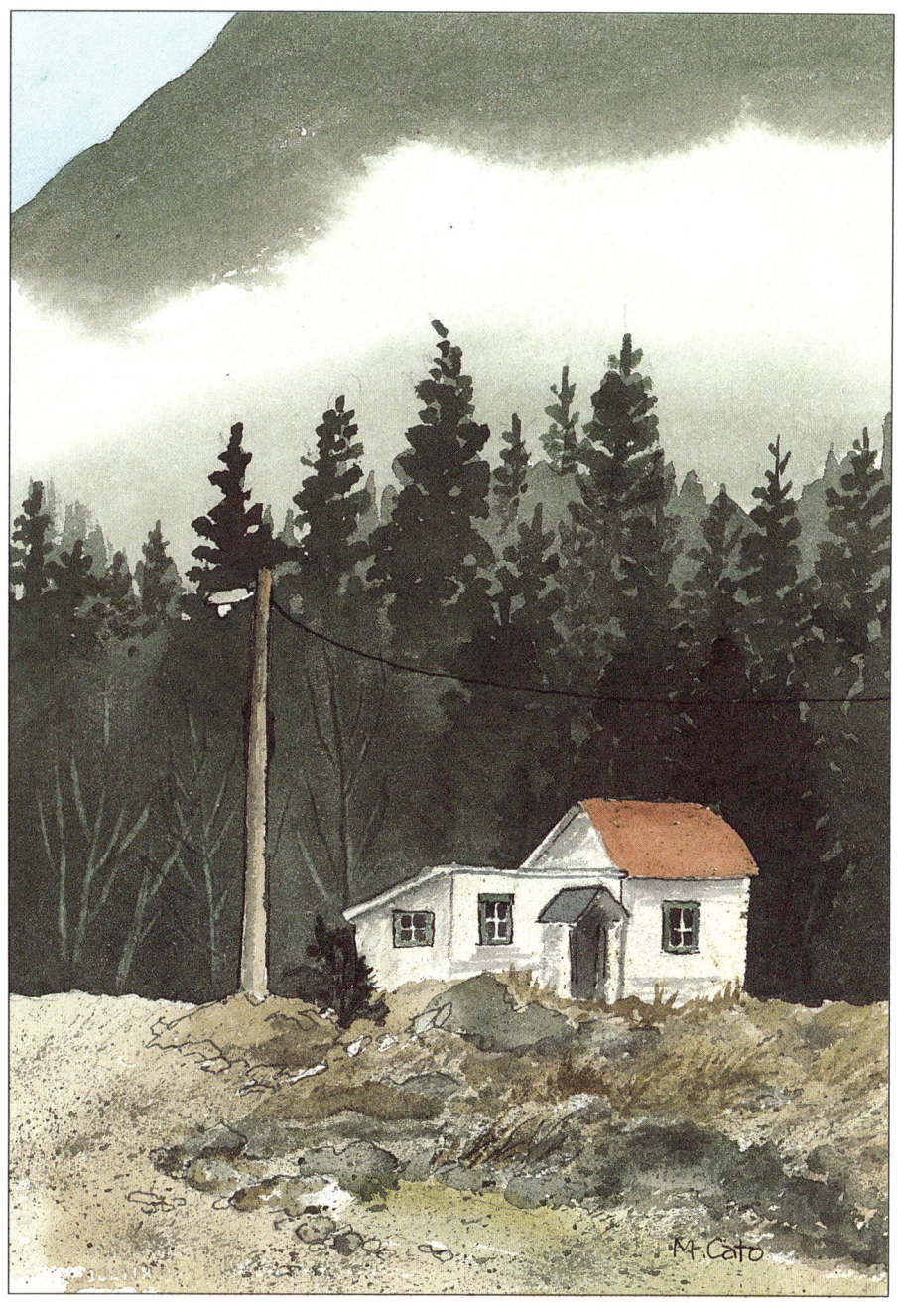

Speakers the next day were Kathy, Jim, Mary, Tom, Pat, Lorraine, Ruth and Gerry. Most expressed a "basic desire...for a richer Christian community life" and described their efforts to be "supportive of and responsive to the needs of the Indian people, both in this rehabilitation project and in the villages." Then Ruth Little "indicated how a family coming here should be prepared to face difficult living conditions and accommodations", which she hoped could be improved.

Life Before and After: Mabel's Story

My first recollection of alcohol was being with my stepfather Willie. He had me on his shoulders and he was calling out for my mother. We looked all over the place for her. Somehow I knew that they had drunk a big amount of home-brew. For as it was brewing in the crock, we smelled it. They would have fun for awhile, then it would turn ugly. We always knew when to run and hide. Just as mom had learned to hide when Willie got violent. Little did I know that he was using me as bait to lure mom back home.

Every Christmas dad John ordered his usual order of a case of Hudson Bay rum, and a case of six gallons of wine. He sat in his chair and drank and drank. It was such a cold lonely feeling! He'd sing for awhile, then he would turn angry. He would kick us out of the house. He held a rifle in our faces and demanded us to leave.

By the time I reached the age of 12 I felt attracted to the booze. It seemed there was some fun in it. It warmed my insides and gave me courage to make friends with the young men in the community. I enjoyed being held and loved.

Then I married at the age of 19, and lived without alcohol in my life. I had three more children after my marriage to Harry. We were happy. Until he started staying out later and later with his work buddies.

I started going out with him on weekends and the alcohol and me made friends once more. It was fun. But Harry couldn't get enough at times and wouldn't bother coming home to the children and me.

When our baby was a year old, Harry walked out on me with another woman. He couldn't forgive me for being unfaithful to him. I had tried to apologize, but to no avail. It turned out she was the wife of the man I had gone out with. Something I chuckle at today.

The separation was painful and I couldn't handle the children crying for their father. I would cry too. The Children's Aid Society helped me make a decision to give the children up for care until I straightened out my act. They were placed in a home together.

My drinking increased with each day as I tried desperately to kill my pain and my guilt. My poor children needed me and I had let them down.

Each day was filled with alcohol, men and pain. Hangovers got steadily worse. I ended up down on Skid Row. Living right with the people I felt happiest with. They never judged me. They just drank as much and as fast as I did.

I lost count of the boyfriends I had. One of them just fresh out of prison taught me the ropes of prostitution. He taught me to use my friendliness and charm to earn us money. The faster I made the money, the faster he spent it on his disease — gambling. He played poker and pool. Of course, as with all my boyfriends, he fooled around on me.

Then I met this man named Joe. He was so much fun to be with. He could talk about things other than what hurt. He could make me laugh. I felt good with him.

One day I walked into the Welfare Office and they introduced me to a new worker. Doreen looked at my file and said, "It says here that you have four children. How often do you see them?" I told her I never ever saw them unless I made an appointment to have them for an afternoon or something.

In about three months Doreen had the ball rolling for me to get one of my kids back. We were going to move slow, as I hadn't had them for about eight years. I forget how long.

I found an apartment in Richmond. Joe and I moved in and we got new furniture through the Welfare. It felt good to have a nice home. At the same time it was scary to think I had to be a mother again. It always hurt me to think that as soon as I was born, my mother walked out on my dad.

Judy came home and it didn't take long to figure out that she was out for revenge. She did everything to go against my wishes. It hurt her because I wasn't with Harry Sr. anymore and she wanted her dad with us.

I drank heavier and heavier and realized that something was definitely wrong in the way I drank. I enjoyed my high and then realized that I needed it. I pulled the wool over my workers' eyes for awhile. Then I got my youngest child back home. Judy had moved out on her own. We just didn't get along anymore.

Finally it caught up with us that it had been noticed that Joe and I drank too much and the Welfare thought we should go for help. I didn't know what we needed help for. If Joe would slow down on his drinking, everything would be OK.

So, we went to a place called Ka Ka Wis on May 7, 1982. What a scary experience. I never knew a place such as this existed and I never knew other people had the same problem. I thought I was the only one. I mean, by the time I admitted something was truly wrong.

We went through the six-week program and then went home. We did fine for awhile. I did fine for four months and had a drink again. I drank for four months. Feeling more and more guilty for what I had done to my son and my Joe. That was so painful!

At the end of February, early one morning I woke up and felt the sun beating down on me. Perspiration poured from every part of my body. I could smell the stench. My heart was beating hard. My joints hurt. In raising my hand to my face I found it glistening with sweat. "By God, Mabel, you're still alive! There's still some life there to salvage!" I yelled out to the Lord: "You said You could help. Well, now is the time!"

It didn't take very long to stand shakily and seek out my son and my Joe. They were washing the dishes in the kitchen as they talked in hushed tones. They knew that if they woke me I would either be in a bad mood, or I'd be out that door like a shot to get another bottle.

"Today is the day. I quit!," I said to them. Then I listed all I would need in my recovery. Lots of soup, cold water, and please not to ask me how I am doing. That I would suffer this out. Never have I seen two happier guys than my son and my Joe. I took two weeks to finally let go of the craving.

We got a call for a job coming up in Ka Ka Wis. And we were so thrilled we went running to the phone, not even thinking to ask our son Harry if he wanted to go with us. Joe and I got the jobs and settled in Ka Ka Wis almost immediately. Harry joined us later.

My hands did things it never used to. I used to be feeling sorry for myself all the time and would make Joe lift things for me. It was so much fun working. The children in the Daycare where I worked were a way for me to renew my flame of motherhood.

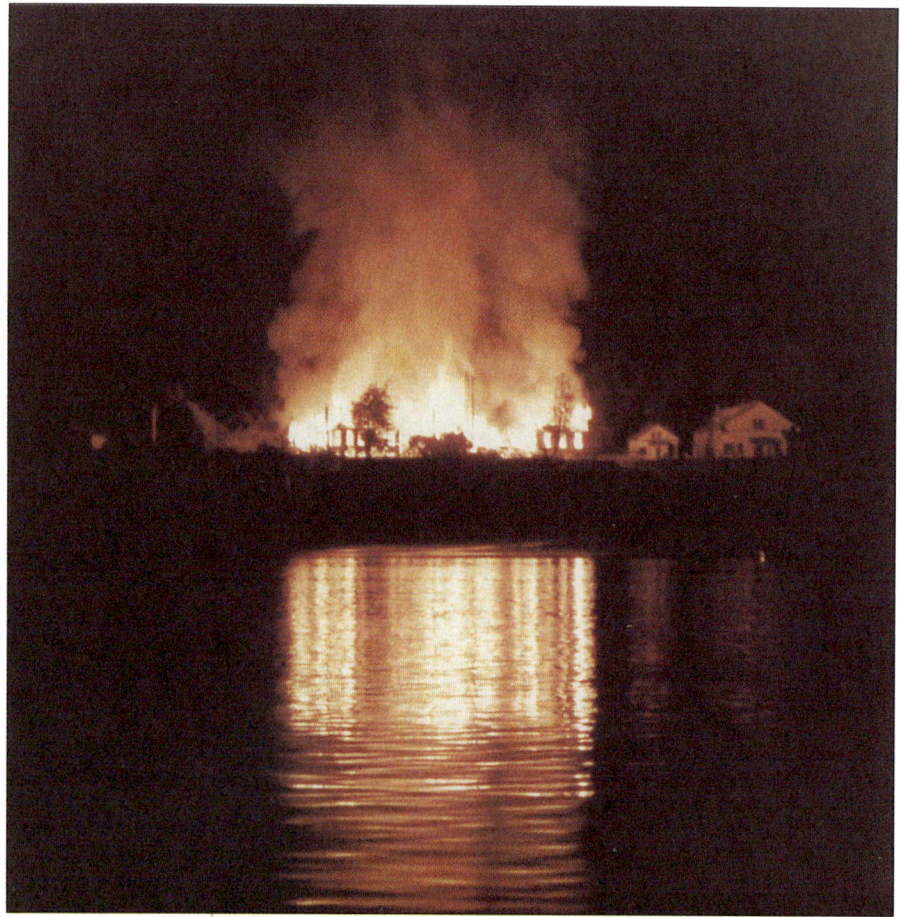

Christie School ablaze in July 1983

My voice came alive once more. Songs came out of my lips as I was putting babies to sleep. My arms could hold and give comfort, whereas before they pushed away people that I loved. Arms that were held out in invitation to true caring, rather than just using a person for my own needs.

Eyes clear to see the beauty of creation. There were times I went to parks and didn't see beauty at all. Mainly a feeling of "Why do I have to waste my time at this dumb park? I want to be in the bar."

Close to the ocean once again. All my childhood I had enjoyed being near water. Dad was a fisherman. How I had longed to be near water again, and here I was in a beautiful place.

Chances were taken. Trust was built once more. There were people here willing to listen to my ideas. I did count!

A gentle push got me writing poetry. It felt weird at first as I had no idea how to do this. But a little voice kept saying that I could do it. In time I developed my own style.

Decisions, choices and plans. Things I was a failure at before, now was a time to try them out. With each one that I accomplished, strength rose within me. Pride was strong. The part that hated like hell being Indian now heard the drums beat loud and clear. My aboriginal name sounded good to me.

In attending potlatches I became aware of how my ancestors carried on traditions. With each year I learned more and more family ties. Now I have a big family. There are hundreds of us. I am no longer lonely.

The fear of being a parent is gone. If my child is unwilling to forgive me for the choice I made two years ago, then that is theirs to deal with. I need not say "I'm sorry" over and over.

If I face something difficult, I feel challenge, and from there I tackle whatever it is. Say it is a new crochet pattern. It may be difficult, but I try. If I can't do it exactly the way it says to, then I will improvise.

The once shy person now stands in front of groups and speaks freely. Loudly and strong. There are many people standing up there with me as I speak. Starting with the stepfather who carried me on his shoulders, right down to the last client who leaves Ka Ka Wis. We work as one here. We learn from one another.

The beauty of change is that I don't say, "Why couldn't I have done this long ago?" I live for today and go with what the Creator has given me. He is my strength.

There is a time for everything to happen. Even a time for the wave to hit the beach. Just as it was exactly the right time for Mabel James to be a drunk, be a wife, be a prostitute, then a time to sober up. No questions. Go with the time.

Change is wonderful. Life is wonderful. It is a voice and it is a tune. It is a gift. Something I will leave for my children and grandchildren. Something I will leave for those yet to come into the world.

Top Priorities: Safety and Health

Improved safety standards and better health safeguards at Ka Ka Wis were the "top priority for action" when the Board of Directors submitted a funding request to the B.C. Ministry of Health early in 1982. The directors' request was backed up by a wide-ranging coalition of aboriginal, civil and religious leaders, Centre staff and volunteers.

"Many of the facilities and much of the equipment we have been using... are old and in need of upgrading," Pat Koreski, then board chairman, wrote to Health Minister J. Nielsen. "In addition our staff is very limited and they are often at the point of exhaustion....Without your advice and financial support we would not be where we are today. We are counting on your continued support."

Other letters also arrived on the health minister's desk. Excerpts:

- From the Nuu-chah-nulth Tribal Council, representing some dozen bands in the western half of Vancouver Island: "It was moved by Larry Baird, Ucluelet Band, that the Tribal Council support Ka Ka Wis Centre to seek funds to upgrade their facilities. Seconded by Richard Lucas. Carried."

- The Clayoquot Band gave an enthusiastic endorsement: "That the Clayoquot Band wholeheartedly support the Ka Ka Wis Family Development Centre. We fully support additional funding for operation and maintenance of the complex. We further resolve that the Ka Ka Wis Family Centre is understaffed and in great need of major repairs, eg. fire fighting equipment, physical safety, health safety, etc. We further resolve that the Centre is a great assistance to many people."
- Dr. Richard G. Foulkes, Board member and administrator of the Tofino General Hospital, confirmed the need for better health and safety standards on Meares Island. He noted that the estimated cost for these requirements was "somewhere between $50,000 and $200,000". This, in his view, was a "modest amount...when compared to the economic and social costs of alcoholism and the revenue generated for the provincial and federal governments from the sale of liquor."
- Father Allan A. Noonan, superior of B.C. and Alberta Oblates, was equally supportive. He and his councillors "wholeheartedly support and encourage the Board in their efforts to make Ka Ka Wis a safer and healthier place to live." The letter noted that the Oblates had supported the program with manpower and funds for 10 years, and also gave the Centre rent-free use of land and buildings.
- Staff and volunteers at Ka Ka Wis hoped for early action to end "the needless anxiety that accompanies our job here....(The) constant concern over the physical safety of clients and staff undermines...energy."
- Simon Lucas, one of the native representatives on the Board of Directors, also sent a letter to the National Native Alcohol and Drug Abuse Program asking for training funds for this "very worthwhile project."

These appeals brought a response from the health minister's office several weeks later. A supplementary grant of $12,000 was approved to purchase essential fire protection equipment. Further funding for upgrading would be taken into account when the department decided the 1982-83 grant to the Centre. When it did arrive, the annual budget grant was $185,914 — nearly $25,000 more than funding granted the previous fiscal year.

30 *Healing Journeys*

The Night Old Christie Burned

Night Fire Destroys West Coast Landmark
Ka Ka Wis to Rise from the Ashes
Spirit Undying - New Trailer Town Replaces Smouldering Ruins

These headlines in July 1983 aptly summarize one of the dramatic turning points in the Ka Ka Wis story.

Dramatic because the flames from that Friday night blaze on July 15 lit up the night sky throughout the Clayoquot Sound region. It was a turning point because the fire totally destroyed a historic landmark — the former residential school building that since 1974 had been home for the Ka Ka Wis counselling program for client families.

Three other buildings also burned to the ground and three families lost all their possessions. Fortunately, no one was hurt. And early fears that the accidental fire might also mean the end of the Family Development Centre were unfounded.

Instead, sixteen 50-ft. trailers, which had been used at a logging camp, were bought from MacMillan-Bloedel and freighted to the Meares Island site, set

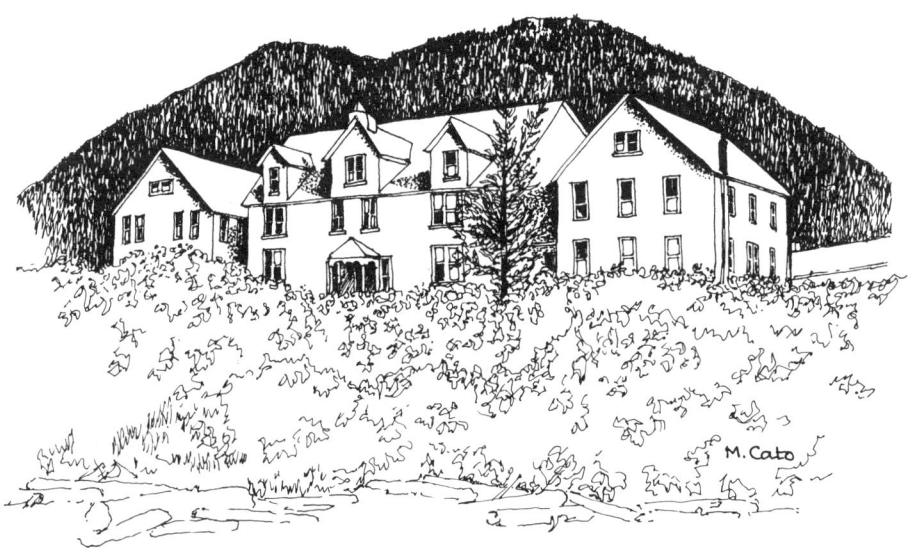

up and outfitted. A round-the-clock team effort meant that only one six-week program session had to be cancelled because of the fire.

"It was great to see the courage and faith" of those who spearheaded the rebuilding project soon after the loss, Sister Margaret Cantwell, SSA, later recalled. "It was little short of miraculous to see the logging trailers arrive and then set up in an area hewn out of the forest."

Several others were so moved by the fiery destruction and rapid reconstruction that they committed their recollections to paper. One was Father Larry Mackey, OMI, once the Christie School principal. From his account of the fire:

"By 4 A.M. nothing was left but a brick chimney that marked the perimeter of where the huge old building stood. Gerry (Guillet) and Reggie (O'Brien) stood looking at the charred ruins and sensed that these ashes were not the end but spoke of a new beginning. The Ka Ka Wis Family Development program had healed too many hearts and broken homes to let it die."

Pat Koreski, Centre administrator, wrote about "The Death of a Friend". Part of his open letter:

"The main building was a centre for learning and sheltered the people dedicated to this pursuit from the storms of the West Coast for 71 years. For the last 10 years it was a centre of Healing. The Healing sometimes of the people who had experienced hurt by the lack of understanding between the two cultures working side by side in the building years before.

"The main building was a creative, well-loved symbol of this ongoing struggle to bring new life to people, all people — students, clients and especially the dedicated staff who ran it as a school and then as a rehabilitation centre, and almost always at little if any financial gain for themselves.

"This is why I have been getting many calls from all over B.C. from people who became sick inside upon hearing of the fire. This is why my eyes tear up when I think of its loss. We see the death of a great old friend. With the grace of God the spirit of this building will rise from its ashes and live on."

As it did. Bob Cato, maintenance staff member, would write in July 1984: "Here we are one year later, having witnessed the rebirth of Ka Ka Wis, stronger and more vibrant than ever."

Children Heal Dark Memories

It's Thursday morning of the fifth week of the therapy program at Ka Ka Wis. At this time, in each of the different circles of adult clients, youth and children, the "Healing of Memories" takes place. A solemn rite surrounds this event. At the Learning Centre references to "healing" and "memories" were given earlier that week. Young people also picked up on the seriousness of the occasion from chance remarks made by older family members and other clients.

The "Healing of Memories" began the day at the Learning Centre. Students brought their chairs to form a circle with the facilitator, as they did other days for guidance discussions. The facilitator held a tray with a number of dark coloured paper circles. These were "memories" and holding one gave each child a right to speak, to be listened to quietly, to be shown respect. After the sharing, each child put the paper circle into a large seashell waiting on the floor in the middle of the group.

* * * * *

This morning a 10-year-old girl, Ann, began the sharing after the facilitator reminded all of the seriousness of the occasion, of the fact that scars remain, but hurts and pain can go. Children point out some of their own scars on arms and legs.

Then Ann told her memory. When she was eight she had become friends with a house painter, had gone into the house to help him painting windowsills. The painter had come in, touched her, sexually abused her. Ann had told no one (instructions from the house painter), but had confided to her mother at the family forgiveness time just the day before at Ka Ka Wis. Ann was in tears as she sobbed out her story and placed her paper circle in the shell.

Norman, an 11-year-old boy, began in a quiet voice to talk about his fears when drinking parties involving his Mom began at home. He shared various incidents at different intervals: his hand being placed on a hot burner when he protested what one of his Mom's drinking partners was doing; of the times he was shut into his bedroom and climbed out of the window to get to

A History in the Making **33**

his Grandma's; of the cases of beer he had seen come into the house when he was waiting for a promised "I'll take you to the movies" — and how in the morning there were empty cases, but no money for the promised movie. Norman had dumped the remaining beer down the sink, and had got yelled at for it. He broke into tears. Later, Norman spoke of one of his Mom's "friends" who was especially mean to the family now that he was no longer Mom's boyfriend. "You'd better have a gun ready," said the rejected friend. "He breaks windows and bothers the whole family," states Norman.

Norman's 9-year-old sister, Gwen, corroborated with nods and sad eyes what her brother was speaking in broken sentences. She added her own: of seeing her Mother being beaten up and lying on the floor. There were memories too of departures in taxis, of men leaving — like her Father, of short stays in Calgary, of the terrorizer catching up with them.

Brian, another 11-year old boy, talked of two uncles coming to his house for a drinking time. The uncles gave money to the children (Brian's brother and sisters). Finally, one uncle gave Brian five dollars. "That's the night he died," sobbed Brian. All the children are moved. Norman got Brian some Kleenex.

Mary, 8-year-old sister of Brian, talked about fights she had seen, of men coming to rape her Mother, of her Mother's cries, of her Dad beating up her Mother on the couch.

Andy, a 6-year-old, nodded in wide-eyed agreement. He took a paper circle and talked about a big boy on his reserve always ready to beat him up.

Ann broke into the quiet that ensued and described the suicide attempt her Mother had made with pills and knives. "I tried cutting my wrists too, because I was so sad, but Tom saw me and took away the knife. He hid all the knives, but I knew where they were.

"Another thing," added Ann, "I have a paralyzed sister I've never seen. She's in a hospital. I want to see her. I want to see her smile and I want to push her wheelchair. My Mom says we'll go next time we have money, but when the money comes she spends it and we don't go." Ann spoke of running away, but she loves her Mom too much to do that.

The session ended with a few exchanges about forgiving each other for slights or hurts in the Learning Centre. Tom and Mary said they still had something to share; however, they wanted to do it on the beach. Facilitator and children, with the shell, matches, and more paper circles (in case others wanted to share additional memories), headed for the rocks in back of the Learning Centre.

Even though the tide was coming in among the crevices, a knobbed and cracked rock provided a suitable spot to gather above the waves. Brian lit a match and all the students formed a windbreak. The "memories" began to burn. Students and the facilitator prayed the "Serenity Prayer" and the "Our Father" — with special emphasis on the forgiveness part.

While the paper circles burned, Tammy held one of the extras and talked about being asked to baby sit. "No one came home for four or six days," she added. "No one in my family believed me when I told them."

Mary talked of her twin who died. Every one had another brief comment, and then another.

Finally, the paper circles were black ashes. The shell was taken to the water. An angry wave turned over the shell. The ashes were gone. The watching children stood in the drizzle between the wind-blown grey sky and grey, restless ocean. The only calm for a brief interlude was in the children's hearts.

Then they turned to celebrate.

— From a presentation to the B.C. Liquor Policy Review Board by Pat Koreski, April 24, 1987. Children's names were changed for the report.

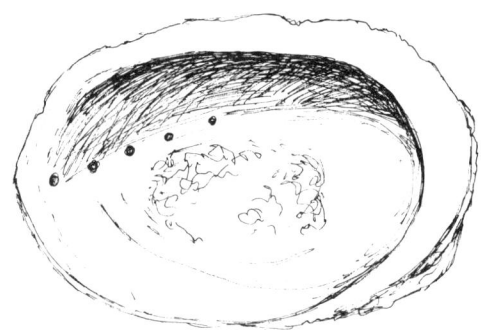

By Maureen Cato

A Celebration of Native Culture

As the boat approaches Ka Ka Wis on Meares Island you may notice off to the right a large arched carving on the height of land where the Christie School had stood. Once ashore you can examine at close range this striking representation of sea and land creatures, fashioned by a gifted native hand.

The outdoor carving has been welcoming clients and visitors since the fall of 1989. Its unveiling that year was announced in a public invitation:

"Nelson & Ruby Keitlah & Family invite you to attend a celebration of new beginnings at Ka Ka Wis Family Development Centre on Saturday, October 21, 1989. This event will be highlighted by the traditional unveiling of new art remembering those who have suffered at the hands of alcohol abuse. Ceremonies will begin at 10.30. Boats will leave Tofino at 9.30."

In its November 22 issue *The Westerly News,* serving readers from Ahousat to Bamfield, featured an account with several photographs. From the report:

"A hundred or so friends and relatives of Nelson and Ruby Keitlah attended a celebration at Ka Ka Wis for the dedication of new art work. Pat Koreski feels that the event 'symbolized the reality that native culture and traditions are alive and strong at Ka Ka Wis.'

"A large carving, which overlooks the ocean, was unveiled on the grounds, and a dozen 8 by 4 ft. art panels were installed in the gymnasium. All the art work, which was commissioned through Ka Ka Wis funding, was designed and created by Vancouver Island native, Cecil Dawson, Ruby Keitlah's son. The art panels were completed with the help of Howard Tom Jr. of Opitsat.

"The ceremonies consisted of a welcome brunch followed by several speeches and the unveiling. Then participants moved into the gymnasium, where cedar boughs decorated the four corners and two ceremonial curtains were employed over the entrances. More speeches, singing and dancing followed, including a new contemporary dance entitled 'The Four Winds', composed by Nelson Keitlah.

"The singing and dancing was followed by traditional gift giving by Nelson, Ruby and Cecil, and then all were invited to close the day with a feast of barbecued salmon, halibut and other specialties.

" 'The whole day was dedicated to the memory of those who have suffered at the hands of alcohol abuse. A strong sense of culture is a strong component in the fight against substance abuse and dysfunctional living,' says Koreski."

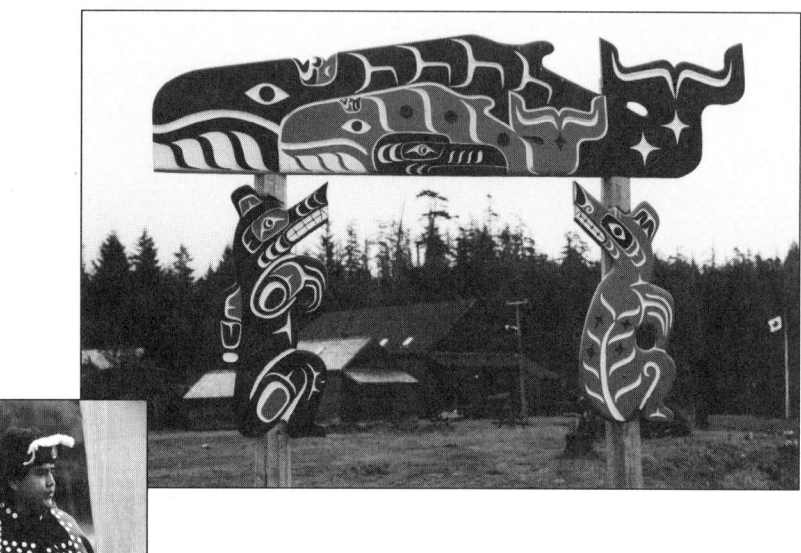

Artist Cecil Dawson

Life and Work on an Island

By P.K.

A big part of the Ka Ka Wis story is living and working on an island, and that means boats. Boats of all sizes and descriptions. It also means big expense and unknown weather conditions from day to day or even hour to hour. This translates into an unique operating style.

A History in the Making   37

The fact Ka Ka Wis is on an island makes for both a romantic, retreat-like atmosphere and at other times for a very scary, isolated feeling. Some staff and clients take to the remoteness and natural beauty very easily, while others find it an annoyance and an inconvenience. A good percentage who find it easy come from homes in similar locations. Other passengers are very afraid of the water.

Being on an island is a built-in deterrent against clients leaving Ka Ka Wis compulsively. The location has served us well in this regard.

In the early years of Ka Ka Wis, two boats used were inherited from Christie School when it closed: the missionary speed boat and the large freight/passenger boat called the "Ave Maria". The "Ave" was a well-known moving landmark around Christie and Tofino. There are many stories and adventures around the "Ave", as it was most often called. "Ave Maria" is Latin for "Hail Mary", the opening words of a very familiar Catholic prayer. This connection seemed to serve the boat well one day early in the 1980's.

Gerry Guillet woke one morning to find the boat missing from its usual mooring out in front of Ka Ka Wis. It had blown hard during the night and was still blowing pretty good in the morning. Gerry and I took the "Remi J.", the 19-ft. speedboat named after our bishop, and began looking for the "Ave". We went out past Vargas Island and back, and then up past "Cluthpitch", the nearby reserve lands and toward the "catface" area. We were beginning to give up hope and expected to see the boat either smashed on some rocks or sunk somewhere. As we started back from "yellow bank", I thought I saw a flash of light, like a mirror, but in the strangest place. We started towards it and as we got closer we could see that it was indeed the "Ave". It had managed to drift past a number of reefs, through a narrow entrance and into a very small bay on the north side of Vargas Island. It had never been in there before. This bay dries up at low tide. The

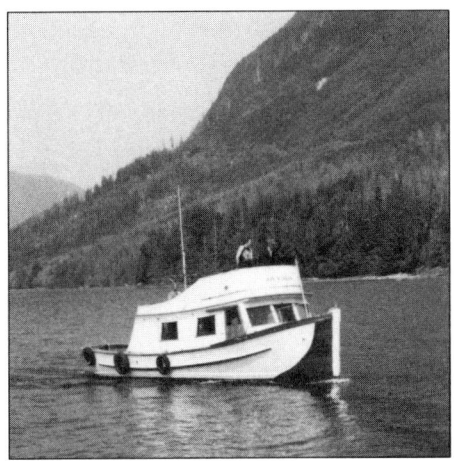

Ave Maria

"Ave" chose the only soft, muddy bank in the bay to come to rest on, and laid peacefully on its side.

I jumped on board and did a quick once over. All looked okay, although the bilge alarm was ringing loudly. I shut off the bell. We waited for the tide to rise and float the old girl once more. When it was floating, we checked for leaks and found none. Soon after floating, I started the engine and slowly navigated the reefs out of there. All was well and we had our boat back. If not a miracle, this was at the least a very special and unusual occurence. No boat ever before or since drifted away from Ka Ka Wis in such an unusual manner and with such a happy ending.

The "Ave" has been sold, thoroughly rebuilt, and is docked at Gabriola Island. It is closer now to its original builder, Barney Williams, Sr., who lives in Nanaimo.

There are many stories and adventures that revolve around Ka Ka Wis and our unusual way of transportation over the years. Many people have been left standing, waiting on the wrong dock for a boat ride, or waiting for the boat at the right dock with the times mixed up, or just waiting. It is always a concern for visitors as to how they are going to get to Ka Ka Wis, once they find it is on an island. And sometimes there is a concern for all passengers when the seas kicks up. But that's another chapter for another day.

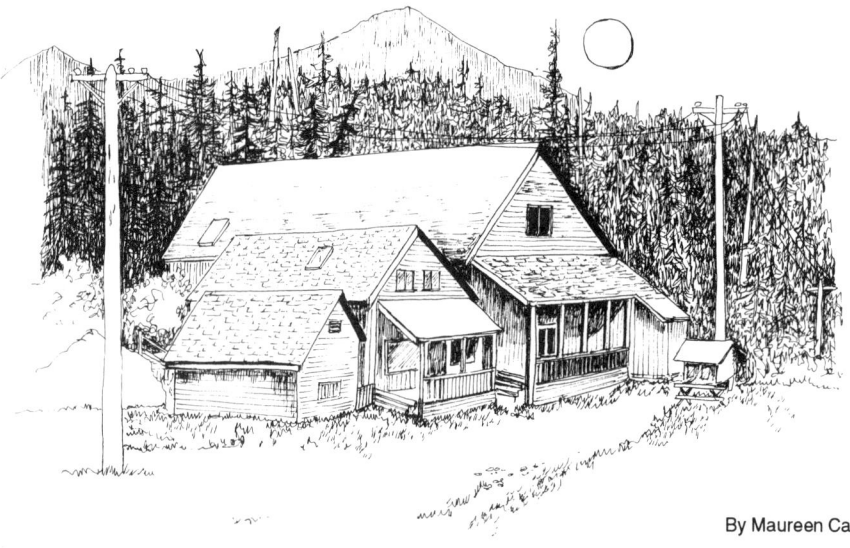

By Maureen Cato

Problem and Solution

There is not enough room to print all the interview reports and clients' comments at hand. So we have made several representative selections from this surplus of grassroots' opinion, and grouped them under these headings: CLIENT VOICES, MEMORIES and REASONS TO CELEBRATE.

Client Voices I: Speaking from the Heart

"Thanks Ka Ka Wis, for giving me that second chance," a native client wrote after taking part in the Centre's counselling program. The writer spoke for hundreds of aboriginal brothers and sisters. Most adult clients who commit to paper their thoughts and feelings about the healing experience at Ka Ka Wis say much the same thing, each in her or his own words: "Thanks for giving me a second chance!"

Heartfelt reflections by clients, written during and after program sessions, are published anonymously in the Centre's newsletter. Here is a first representative sampling of what adults, youth and children have shared through the pages of the *Ka Ka Wis Star* since it began publishing in 1983, and in other Centre sources.

- "I'd lost my wife and lost my kids. I was living all by myself. My children came to my house and asked me if I could come to Ka Ka Wis with them. I realized that they still had that love for me and that I had love for them, so I came. At first it was hard for me as an alcoholic and drug addict. In the third week I just about left. Just so afraid, sweating....But I stayed for the six weeks and I'm glad I did."

- "I thought Ka Ka Wis was just for alcoholics, but I was wrong. I came here to support my husband with his drinking problem. Little did I know that I needed help too. There were so many problems I had hidden...especially my anger."

- A boy writes: "When I see an eagle flying above me, I know that my grandpa is watching over me and letting me know I'm going to be safe for today."
- A wife and mother writes to her husband: "We've come a long way. Some days were hard, some were easy. But the day we stood in church and my father gave me away, we said our 'I do's.' We really toughed it out and I'm happy about that. Thank you for four beautiful children. Happy anniversary. All my love and friendship."
- A client remembers:
  "Ka Ka Wis
  A place of learning.
  Almost 20 years ago I left here,
  Figuring I'd never return for learning,
  Only to find I am returning
  For even more and more learning."
- "All I've seen are women crying. Men should cry too. Letting it stay inside you only hurts more. Don't be afraid to shed tears. You only teach your children to hold back feelings too. Sure they'll get scared, but if you tell them why, they will understand you. Sure they're small, but they do have brains, and when you think of it, they are very smart."
- "We don't have to cry in our beer anymore. We can cry on our loved one's shoulder. We can also learn not to have anything to cry about."
- A family man makes a new start: "I have done a lot of things and seen a lot in my life. Now with new eyes open and new feelings, soon I will be beginning a real strong and loving future....With God's guidance and strength I will become a better man when I finish. I will carry my bluebead with me always to remind me of my friends who have shared inner thoughts, pain and happiness. You all have helped me find the real me. I thank you all with all my heart and soul."
- "We are heading out into the real world again. With a different outlook on each of our lives. Taking with us new tools...and putting them to great use. I will put great effort into a better, sober life, with a better understanding and without shame."

- "I will miss Meares Island and its beauty. Lone Cone. The ocean and waves. Trees, squirrels, raccoons, the birds. The wolves that roam the dark nights, heard but not seen. The wind that seems to whisper the great spirits into our being. Spirits that give us much hope, serenity, peace, security, love, and wisdom to respect and care about our traditions and culture...."
- "I hope I can find another Ka Ka Wis out there in the concrete jungle."
- "May you find within yourselves your own little Ka Ka Wis on embarking on your new life from here. May you also walk hand in hand with the Creator."
- I see that I have been given a reprieve by God in the form of caring people. I have been given a chance to live again — one day at a time."

Memories of the Early Years

The pioneer spirit that characterizes new settlements and new ventures certainly was evident during "the growing-up years" at Ka Ka Wis. The vivid memories of Centre pioneers describe the exhilarating and sometimes anxious 10 years when native and white partners shared a common goal, trusted one another and the Higher Power, and, despite long odds, by determined co-operation made their dream come through. Some of the many memories recalled during 1993 interviews:

- When Old Christie closed, one former student, by then the father of a large family, was preoccupied "with the need to use the school buildings for our people". Louie Frank was already convinced some sort of treatment program at Ka Ka Wis would be the best way "to come to grips with the alcohol problem....Some of us saw the potential at Christie and we saw that somebody had to get the ball rolling...."
- Barney Williams Sr. was another aboriginal leader who had the same hope. "Over 20 years ago I wrote a letter to each of the chiefs along the coast asking them to support the Ka Ka Wis program when it started. I said alcoholism was our biggest problem. I saw that the Centre could be a stepping stone. Then other steps could follow." The native elder, now in his late

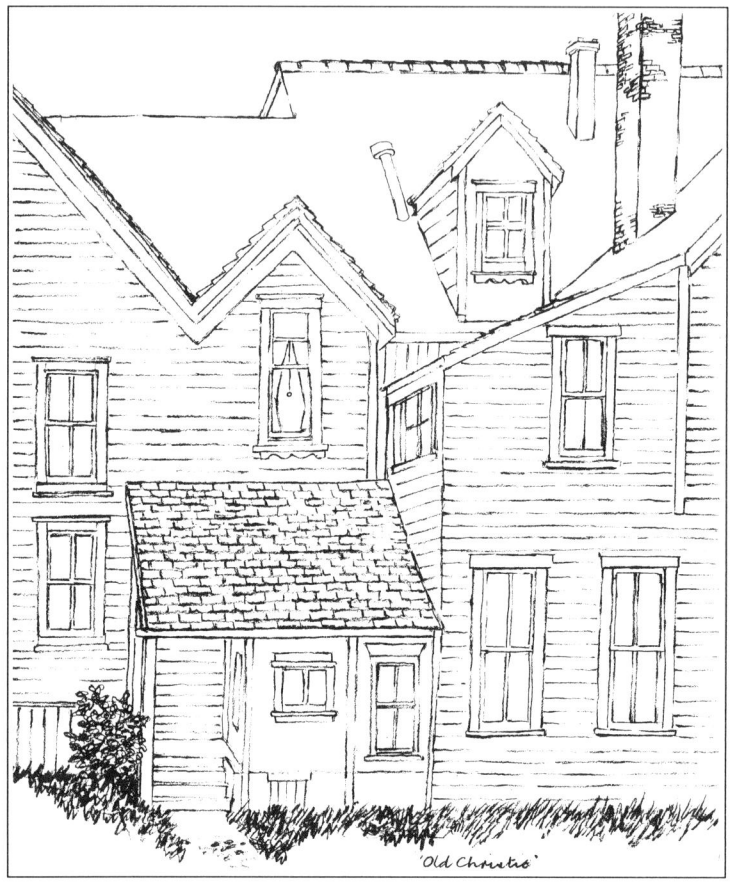

'Old Christie'

By Maureen Cato

70's, who still likes to captain a seine boat, added: "I hope Ka Ka Wis will stay there for a long time to come. I know for sure from many people who went there that it's done a lot of good."

- United Church missionary Lloyd Hooper, friend and colleague of Gerry Guillet, recalled that they used to visit west coast native communities together, sometimes sharing the same mission boat. "The native people made us aware of the need to do something about alcoholism. They just said, 'We need help!' Gerry and I were determined to keep close to them in what they wanted."

- The Oblate priest agreed that "the idea really came from the grassroots. It was the dream of the native people.... The Spirit was moving the people."

A History in the Making **43**

- Reg O'Brien said the opening of the new Family Development Centre was "a great turn of events" that in time would help "many hurting people."
- But once founded, Ka Ka Wis experienced some precarious early years, Jim MacDonell, OMI, the first director, pointed out. "All in all, there were the good times and the not so good. The physical labour involved was often at the breaking point. We had all this plus the new program to maintain. There was a Higher Power at the helm, for sure. Otherwise, it would have been impossible."
- "It really feels good to take a walk down memory lane," said Lorraine LaMarre, SSA, the Centre's first senior counsellor, when recalling her Ka Ka Wis years of 1973-81. Sometimes, admittedly, "it was quite discouraging and lonely — just the isolation of the place. The work was physically difficult. And we were disappointed when some of the first people who came for counselling soon were drinking again. It really was a question of survival those first few years. But we hung in there."
- In 1974 John Lucas came on his own to Ka Ka Wis for counselling and stayed almost a year. "It worked out pretty good but it took awhile," he said in describing his struggle with alcohol. "I helped out with the work — clearing areas, cutting wood, repairing buildings."
- Alban and Rose Michael were one of two native couples who lived at Ka Ka Wis for several months in 1973-74. Rose helped in the community kitchen while Alban worked on the landing float. "I felt at peace there," Rose Michael said. "I felt comfortable with the people there. I was sorry to leave."
- "Nothing can take away the small success stories," Kathy Erickson/Seitcher stressed in reviewing her more than 10 years at the Centre, beginning in 1973. "These stories show that the human spirit can overcome addiction, often permanently. More than that, lots of families recover their family spirit at Ka Ka Wis." Kathy recalled the encouraging advice the pioneer staff received from Victoria psychiatrist Dr. Iain Kenning: "When a person is free for even one day from any addiction, that's an accomplishment. And six weeks at Ka Ka Wis without alcohol or drugs is cause to celebrate."
- "It was quite a struggle," Brother Tom Cavanaugh, OMI, said in describing the "many ups and downs" the Centre staff experienced in the 70's. "But see what a beautiful thing is happening there now!"

- "I found it so relaxing after hospital administration work," Mary McGarrigle, SSA, remembered. " It really was a community of love. The Saint Ann sisters and the Oblates had their separate houses but we came together for suppers and prayers. Sometimes native families came to visit. We played cards, we sang, we had a good time...even though we didn't have much. I did a lot of the cooking. I loved it there."

- Marjorie Kuntz, a registered nurse, also has happy memories of her few years on Meares Island in the mid-'70's. "Coming straight from Toronto, I was struck by the serenity of the place and amazed by the people on staff.... by their easy acceptance of everything."

- "Just the fact that they kept going is cause to celebrate," observed Patricia Donovan, SSA, referring to the earlier Centre team before she joined them in 1976. "We can be thankful that they did not give up in those early days despite all the hardships they had to deal with." And what about her contribution to the team effort in her four years there? "I was doing a lot of the nitty-gritty background jobs, paper work and other details," replied this self-named "Martha".

- When preparing a taped memoire of their Ka Ka Wis years Pat Donovan and Jim MacDonell referred to the " great asset" Ray Williams had been while at the Centre over a period of several years. An early client, he became a versatile helper on several fronts, Patricia reported: "Besides maintenance, he did counselling in the AA program. He was also good in outreach to native communities....He liked to listen and talk to people." Jim added, "He was a great mechanic who could fix almost anything."

- The Andrew family — Wilfred, Margaret and their children from Friendly Cove, lived and worked at Ka Ka Wis from 1978 to 1985, longer than any other native couple. Margaret said: "Staying there all those years and going through every program made me really look at myself. Every time we did the AA readings about the 12 Steps, I saw them in a different way and they told me a new thing about myself and life."

- Virginia Vandean/LeJeune was the first classroom teacher at Ka Ka Wis in 1977-78. She recalled the way older sisters and brothers helped younger native siblings at the new Learning Centre. Eleven children from one family were in her care during one program session. "One little girl of around 10 could not read when she came but after six weeks she could read grade one books. She was so excited about being able to read that she carried the book around with her." Mrs. LeJeune received a minimum salary, some of which she spent for classroom supplies — a fact contemporaries later recalled.

- Don McGinnis, Tofino businessman and veteran member of the Ka Ka Wis Board, emphasized the Centre's modest beginnings. "Nobody was there for the money in those early days. It was 100 per cent dedication." The new program was "running on a shoe string" and the pioneer staff "worked at a survival level". He described one early occasion when Jim MacDonell met with 50 to 80 chiefs and elders of coastal tribes as well as leading Tofino citizens. Martin Saxey, who had been chief baker and boatman at Christie School, prepared "gallons of salad and baked beans" for the event. "Jim laid out what the Centre hoped to accomplish. The meeting agreed that the idea sounded viable."

Reasons to Celebrate

During dozens of interviews natives and members of the majority culture alike listed many reasons why the Ka Ka Wis experience should be celebrated. Some of the comments heard, mostly from persons familiar with the Centre's pioneer years:

- Gerry Guillet credits the Spirit of God, aboriginal leaders and an unnamed native couple "who drank themselves to death" for the dream that became a reality when Ka Ka Wis Centre was born. "The process started at Kyuquot where some native leaders took the alcohol problem seriously and wanted to see Old Christie used for family programs. But without the few key people who were keeping the old place going — Jim and Reg, Lorraine and Kathy — the program would never have got started."

Then Gerry described the earlier contribution made by the couple he did not name. "Once he said to me, 'Padre (he always called me that), why don't you ...make a centre out of Old Christie for people like me and my wife so we can go there for treatment and bring the family with us?'

"I always remembered him saying that because within a few months both parents were dead. When she died he was devastated. He drank himself to death within a month. What a shame that they died from drink. Yet I don't think they died in vain. Ka Ka Wis came about for people like them and partly, I think, because of them. The sacrifice of their death was not wasted. That young couple were the ones who made me follow the promptings of the Spirit....

"Even if one person or family sobered up at Ka ka Wis and saved their life, that would be reason enough to celebrate. In fact hundreds of families and individuals have been brought back to sobriety and new life. Thank God!"

- Lorraine LaMarre, SSA, now a senior adviser at her religious order's Mother House in Quebec, celebrates for the same reasons Gerry gave and many others. "I celebrate that the idea of a family centre came from the native people themselves....I celebrate that I helped to bring this dream to birth and helped nurture it during its infancy and childhood. I celebrate that together we made many people aware of the importance of bringing the whole family to Ka Ka Wis for counselling. I celebrate that Ka Ka Wis was the first such centre in North America, and one of the first anywhere."

After citing further reasons to celebrate, she summed up: "I celebrate all the people who ever were at Ka Ka Wis — the people who worked there and the people who came there. It was a real team effort from the beginning!"

- Louie Frank is thankful he, Eva and their children moved to Ka Ka Wis the first year the program was being organized. "We just wanted to make the point that this thing could be done. We stayed a whole year. We were fortunate to be there with the people who were there."

The aboriginal leader never mentioned the problems the Frank family had at Ka Ka Wis with freezing living quarters, a baulky stove, and the long hours he spent each school day boating his children to and from Tofino for classes. Instead, he emphasized that he continues to celebrate the Ka Ka Wis reality.

- Reg O'Brien, the Oblate veteran, celebrates that Ka Ka Wis has "helped a lot of hurting people", many of whom he first knew as Christie School students. "It's amazing, really. In spite of all the negative things that come up about the old residence, you'll notice that most natives like to come back here." This in itself is cause enough to celebrate for the man whom Gerry Guillet describes as the "living thread that runs through the whole story" of Ka Ka Wis. "Reg is a good listener and has a quiet way of counselling. He has helped a lot of people over the years."

- Board member Don McGinnis sees "lots of reasons" to celebrate. "I can't think of one person who left Ka Ka Wis, either as a client or as staff, who did not appreciate the experience, the opportunity of having been there." Moreover, "I think Ka Ka Wis has been a benefit to this whole west coast, not only for the many client families. I know it works."

- Ray Williams spent more than four years at Ka Ka Wis on an on-and-off basis in 1974-81 — sometimes as a client, always as a versatile helping hand in both maintenance and counselling. " How do I feel when I look back on those years? Well, I feel a sense of accomplishment for my people as well as for your people. Ka Ka Wis is helping out everybody."

- Kathy Erickson/Seitcher, now director of the Port Alberni Drug & Alcohol Counselling Service Society, celebrates the Ka Ka Wis staff's successful struggle to survive in the Centre's early years. "And I celebrate Larry Mackey. He kept pushing us, telling us, 'It's a great idea. You can do it!'"

  She is thankful too for the tireless support given the new counselling team by the aboriginal families who came to live at Ka Ka Wis — the Franks, the Michaels, the Littles, the Williams, the Girvans and the Andrews.

  Another reason to celebrate is that "Mother Nature is slowly reclaiming the old school site. We never used to see deer or eagles there in the '70's. Now you do, plus wolves and bears."

- Janis McDougall, teacher at the Learning Centre in 1978-80, celebrates "the retreat environment" on Meares Island. "That environment is something to celebrate because of the way it helps so many families."

- Ka Ka Wis has been and is still making "a great difference" in the lives of hundreds of west coast native families. Frank Salmon, OMI, celebrates this achievement which the missionary priest to west coast tribes has witnessed first hand since 1976.

"Living in Ahousat and visiting the other villages for 17 years, I can see the good results probably better than most people. Ka Ka Wis isn't the only factor but it has had a real impact on attitudes towards drinking on the reserves. And I can also say that the Centre's emphasis on family development has helped a lot of couples."

Former Ka Ka Wis clients who have maintained sobriety "are the core of the AA groups" in several native communities, he reported. In Ahousat, the largest aboriginal community on the coast, local support groups are growing. "Every time another couple completes the Ka Ka Wis program there is a big meal put on by some local people. Every New Year's we have sober dances. And sober house parties are arranged throughout the year. Every sports day used to be a time of heavy drinking. Now that's just about gone. The picture is really turning around."

Poems I: The Laureate of Ka Ka Wis

She came for awhile, went away, then returned. First she came as a client who had survived incest, family breakup and alcoholism. Later she shared her mothering skills at the Ka Ka Wis Toddlers' Learning Centre (day care). Nowadays this aboriginal grandmother is an experienced counsellor of adult clients.

She also writes poems. In fact Mabel James is "Poet Laureate" at Ka Ka Wis. Since she first arrived she has written dozens of poems, and sometimes prose pieces. Many have been published in the Centre's newsletter. Verses from three of her works:

Let It Fall

("Dedicated to my best friend Joe Kubota....When I was drinking, I wore many masks. The one I wore the most was of anger. Then one day, I met someone I could act myself with. Today I wish to thank Joe for helping me find my own personality." - M.J. July 25, 1986)

This mask I hide behind
Living, and paying no mind
To what really matters to me —
Through false eyes I see....

Appearing to be so strong —
Like nothing is really wrong.
Making like I can do it alone,
Independence is always shown.

Like I don't need a friend,
Different relationships I end.
Another thing I hide
So deep inside....

Is the loneliness,
The emptiness,
The want of people all around,
Laughter to me is a haunting sound.

Then one day it did change —
It felt ever so strange!
I gave up all —
And let the mask fall.

Ka Ka Wis

A mountain behind her does stand
And cool waters skirt her land.
Trees so green and so tall —
And God created them all.

No busy traffic for me to hear.
Just quiet, and air so clear.
A beach so big with lots of sand —
All numbered by our Creator's hand.
Winds that blow ever so strong,
Storms that don't last too long.
He shows His strength in all of these.
And his gentleness in whispering trees....

Memories you will leave behind.
A better road now you'll find.
Brothers and sisters, remember this;
You learned to walk again at Ka Ka Wis.

Inner Suitcase

(Mabel James offers parting advice to client families as they prepare to return home.)

*You've probably packed most everything
Of all the things you'll bring.
Folded neatly in suitcases
Crowded in some places.*

*Let me help pack this one —
Together we'll make it fun.
Pack it slow and with love.
Ask for help from above.*

*Remember the walks
And talks.
The dinners together
The lousy weather!*

*Place them tenderly inside —
Don't let anything hide.
Pack them all away
For some rainy day.*

*Pack the gifts you cannot see,
Happiness and laughters of glee.
Handle them with care
Now leave them there....*

*Now when you are far away
And you have a lonely day,
Unlock the case and start
Unpacking memories from your heart.*

The Evolving Program

Philosophy and Mission

By P.K.

Our philosophy, loosely put, has been to respond to people's need to change, especially the families' need to do so. We respond in a caring and sharing way, with spirituality as the guiding force. People walk with people in this process of change. Ka Ka Wis provides the space and time for this to happen, but each individual and family ultimately makes it happen or not happen.

Our mission has been to bring about the healing of past and present hurts felt by native families. This is done, first of all, in the context of promoting and supporting sobriety for families caught in the trap of substance abuse, whether it's alcohol or other drugs. Then together we begin to deal with all the other issues that are present.

An official philosophy was adopted by the Board of Directors in the mid 1980's and then slightly modified in the early '90's. In light of new information on addictions, family and community systems and the process of healing, I believe it would be good for the Board and staff to update this statement.

The Centre statement of philosophy as it now reads:

"We of the Ka Ka Wis Family Development Centre Society are dedicated to a holistic approach to individual/family healing and growth. We believe in the intrinsic value of each human being and that every individual has the power of healing within.

"We strive to provide physically, emotionally, mentally, socially and spiritually the environment in which each person and family can respond to and experience their goodness, thus recognizing their potential and making positive and definite choices that will enable them to cope better with life's challenges.

"We believe alcoholism to be a chronic, progressive and often fatal individual/family disease. Its progress and results can and must be controlled and healed within the individual.

"We believe in the healing power of the Circle as guided by the energies of our Higher Power as viewed by us. We believe recovery from substance abuse and other addictions is a lifelong process."

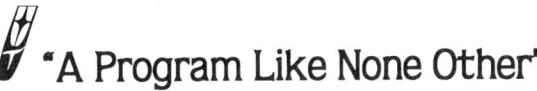 "A Program Like None Other"

By P.K.

Over the years the scheduled program at Ka Ka Wis has evolved, adapted and changed many times. But in truth it isn't the schedule for sessions or any other determined set of exercises that makes Ka Ka Wis different. Really, it is who comes to Ka Ka Wis and what they do while here that makes us unique.

Families, and sometimes extended families, come to live here, formerly for six weeks and now for four weeks. The families come in pain as a result of years, and sometimes generations, of unhealthy choices. Each member of a hurting family is deeply affected by this pain, and each member has an opportunity while here to work at turning this pain around, and so helping the whole family to become much more healthy. The family as a whole and each individual member is invited to make choices that will bring more happiness and less hurt.

The environment at Ka Ka Wis is the key to allowing the program to work. The physical beauty and strength provided by the sea, the creeks, the lake, Lone Cone Mountain, the woods and the beach cannot be overestimated. Also, the absence of TV, the limitation on telephone calls and VHFs (radio phones), the lack of stores and neighbours also provide a dimension that should not be underestimated. And then there are the staff members - a blend of natives and non-natives, those recovering and those non-addicted, academics and non-academics, with families and without, from different backgrounds and cultures. All of them are first and foremost committed to walking with the families who come looking for a better life.

Families provide for their physical needs while at Ka Ka Wis. The cooking, the laundry, the cleaning, and many of the free-time activities are all done in individual family units. This allows families the opportunity to put into practice needed changes, and so experience the wonderful feeling of healthy living.

This living and doing while learning is what enhances and solidifies the different scheduled exercises that families take part in while at Ka Ka Wis. Some of these exercises are centred around what a family is and how it functions. Some are communication exercises, such as communication blocks and postures.(*) There is family mapping, and also the family-roles skit, plus "shoulds and shouldn'ts". Some exercises centre around sensing one's feelings and sharing these feelings. Other exercises focus on past pain and grief, and how to begin letting go of these negatives. The rock exercise and the healing of memories are such exercises. Some activities are spiritually centred, such as the smudging ritual, the sweat-lodge experience, the Circle and the like, as later described.

But whether the environment changes or the various things done here change, the one unique permanent quality of Ka Ka Wis is whole families experiencing together, right away, the change they came here seeking. The goal is that their Ka Ka Wis experience will be strong enough to encourage family members to keep on making positive choices.

The Current Program

By David Zryd, M.A., Program Co-ordinator

To describe what happens during a typical session at Ka Ka Wis is difficult because our program is evolving and changing to meet clients' needs at any given time; it is "client centred" in the true sense of the word. Even though there is a core set of experiential exercises, how those sessions are run also tends to vary because each counsellor brings his or her own personal strengths and beliefs to the group.

The current program is the result of many years of blending, borrowing, and creating group sessions that will reach our clients deeply. Basically, exercises and topics that make a difference and are accepted by the clients are kept. Other ideas are dropped, and still other ideas are recycled from earlier times. Although we at Ka Ka Wis are sometimes hesitant about changing some old stand-by sessions ("If it works, don't fix it!"), the recent move to a shorter four-week program has caused all staff to take a hard look at what is the core of our program.

Before I spell out what we do, I would like to give examples of who the clients may be who come to Ka Ka Wis to join our circle. As you have already read elsewhere in the book, our program is unique in that we serve families — all kinds of families, including single moms or single fathers, blended or intact families, extended families with grandparents, couples expecting children, and occasionally a single person with a support person who lives with that family.

Ka Ka Wis primarily serves Vancouver Island clients, about half of whom are West Coast residents. We also take a few families from other regions of British Columbia. While our program is for the native population, it is not uncommon to have some non-native clients who are married into the main families we serve. The flavour of each session depends on who is in the circle, and this can change depending on where people come from — city, country or reserve around the province.

It is important to note that our distinctive role in the British Columbia Alcohol and Drug Programs is to help client families who are missing some of the supports other families (who do not need our services) may have in their community, such as a steady income, supportive social circle, or a proven ability to maintain sobriety and raise a family in a healthy environment.

One thing all clients have in common is that they are suffering directly or indirectly from the abuse of alcohol or drugs and would like help in recovering. Most often their past includes a history of physical, emotional or sexual abuse. Often the problem stems from past generations of substance abuse, and a neglect of parenting that has caused some clients to grow up largely on their own, or with others in the community who helped out.

It must also be noted that for most of this century residential schools were a part of the experience of being an aboriginal person. In some cases, this time away from home was a great opportunity to learn and better one-

56 *Healing Journeys*

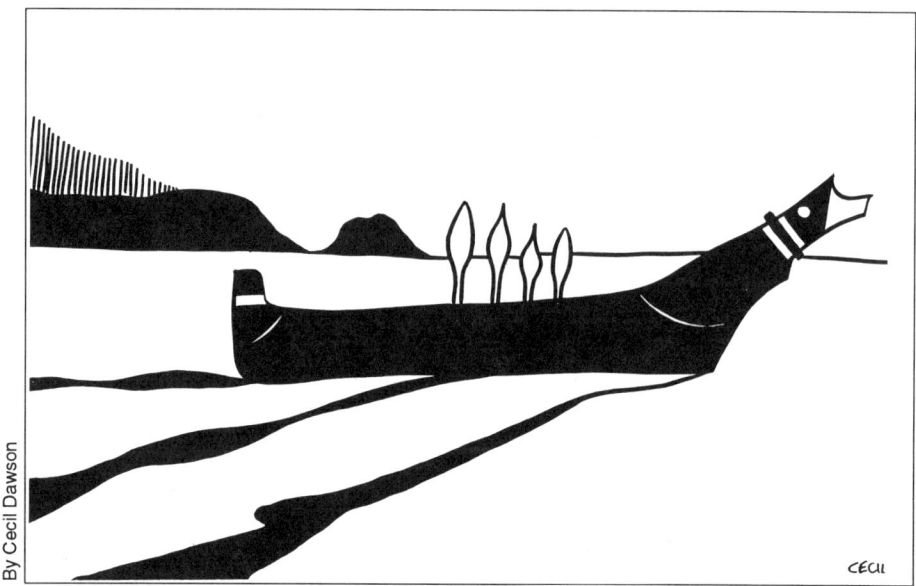

By Cecil Dawson

self; in other cases, residential school was demoralizing and hurt the individual's sense of self-worth and pride in being a native. In most cases being away at school prevented the parents from transferring traditional culture and parenting skills to their children. Many of our clients are either the product of the residential school system, or as children were affected by the system, and now have a legacy of poor parenting skills, made worse through later substance abuse.

Given the need for a program to promote healthy living in a family without alcohol or drug abuse, and with the encouragment to become one's personal best, our program was developed to help heal the memories of the past, while also learning new skills to improve relationships between family members and communities as a whole.

Except for the isolation, client families live at Ka Ka Wis as they would at home. After settling into the living units and adjusting to their new surroundings, the problems left over from earlier times resurface, and old habits that die hard begin to trouble the families again. What's different this time is the opportunity for families to work things out with the staff and other clients in a safe, supportive environment.

For example, a common family problem is being able to go out together and enjoy a fun activity, such as walking on the beach or playing volleyball at the gym. Simple everyday activities like these can be painful for some clients who try to relax and enjoy themselves, only to discover their own painful memories don't include family fun. After working through and grieving for a lost childhood, adult clients finally let go. This opens up new chances to learn and practice family enjoyments they can share when back in their own community.

Another example of experiential healing that happens at Ka Ka Wis is when former residential school students at Christie are once again in the same place to which they may not have returned for 30 or 40 years, and now are flooded with feelings and recollections from their childhood. Clients with issues rooted in their school years at Christie now have the chance to walk the old grounds and begin to resolve any conflicts that still bother them from those earlier days. Strong feelings and commitment to family unity often replace the sense of loss and abandonment they may have felt as a child. For others, returning to Ka Ka Wis is like returning home to an old friend. Memories are kind and there is strength, especially spiritual strength, in being once again in this special place.

Alongside everyday sessions in program, whether it is looking at family roles in a staff skit, struggling with communication-block exercises, or learning to recognize, accept and share your feelings as a family, an unmistakable cultural awareness also is present. For some clients, learning cultural practices is a new experience, for others a rediscovery, and for the elders in session this provides a chance to add something unique and meaningful to the circle.

Cultural practices that have been adopted nationally by First Nations people, such as smudging and the sweat lodge, are balanced with local West Coast customs like traditional songs and drumming. Overall, the rituals bring an appreciation of hospitality and spirituality to everyday life. It is wonderful to witness clients rediscovering their pride of heritage and speaking in their native tongue prayers that were discouraged in an earlier age.

A good example of how Ka Ka Wis celebrates renewed family values is the Blue Bead Ceremony. Other family members come to share and support the individual families who have completed the program. The agenda on Blue Bead Day varies with the desire of each client circle.

No two four-week sessions are the same. But always we cover our main topics, including building relationships, the letting go and healing of painful memories, ways of learning new tools to communicate better and support one another, expressing feelings, and rediscovering one's family tree and cultural practices. These recovery goals are unlikely to change in the near future.

Another part of our program is more flexible and reflects what different client families ask for. Issues like sexuality, sexual abuse, residential-school healing, domestic violence, and suicide are examples of experiences that can and do receive extra time and attention when group concern is expressed.

As a program, we try our best to "walk with" our clients, building trust and working through the issues as they present themselves. Ka Ka Wis gives families an opportunity to "take stock" of where they are on the road of life, and take from our services some "tools" to help in their recovery process. In this sense, the program does not try to be "a fix" to all things, but rather a time to build self-esteem before heading back to everyday life and its many challenges.

Quality Assurance

By George Atleo, counsellor

Much has been said about the program for clients who come to Ka Ka Wis. To provide a program that meets the needs of people from all communities, changes have to be made from time to time. For example, a four-week program versus a six-week program is debatable. However, keeping in mind that our goal is to provide a "Quality Assurance" program for clients, a number of options were looked at. We looked at the underlying program concepts with this assurance of quality as our goal.

1. Community support workers. Are the Ka Ka Wis clients in a recovery program of achieving sobriety? Are they "detoxing"? Are they involved with

a community support group, and are they assessing and planning their program before entering Ka Ka Wis? These are some of the questions we wanted to start working with along with the support workers in the field, so as to provide a good program for clients.

2. For the staff. It is challenging to take care of any personal issues that we as staff have when these concerns are triggered or brought up by clients' issues. Staff training and wellness are designed to meet these personal needs as well as the needs of the whole program. Also, staff training is designed to equip staff with skills to meet the needs of all areas of the program. In this way we are able to rotate our services when called upon, both in the communities and at Ka Ka Wis.

3. The Board of Directors. They have to be involved with all the changes that are happening in the Ka Ka Wis program. It is all of us in partnership, working together to provide a good program for everyone. Working for healthy individuals in healthy families in healthy communities in a strong culture. Everyone is equal. Everyone has taken a personal responsibility to help assure that together we are building a strong future for our communities.

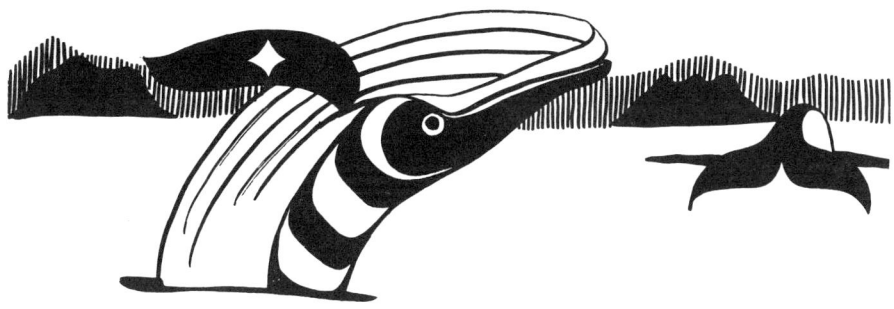

By Cecil Dawson

The Silent Crew

By P.K.

Oftentimes it's the quiet ones who get the job done but receive little recognition. Our maintenance staff easily fits into this category. This involves a long list of individuals over the years.

In the early years, of course, maintenance was largely done by anyone on hand who had a few moments to spare. Ray Williams, Wilf Andrew, Gerry Guillet and Jim MacDonell very often doubled in both program and maintenance in order to help out Reg O'Brien.

Then there were the days of Bob Cato and Joe Hnasiewich giving Reg a hand to keep things going. These were the days of large renovation projects and lots of activity in and around the building, dock and grounds. Howard Johnston doubled in the maintenance and evening attendant routines.

In recent years we have had the quiet presence of Daryl Blackbird and Dave Frank — two of the most self-effacing of the bunch, and to whom the opening sentence most applies. George Atleo shared in this capacity when he first came here, then went mainly into program delivery, where he is the quiet presence.

The support staff often also fill in as ex officio counsellors. Many times the clients reach their limit in session, especially the men, and they seek out a sympathetic ear. Reg and Dave Frank perhaps have the best ears, but all of the maintenance staff fill this function often enough.

Other workers over the years have helped keep the place and boats going. Names such as Tom Johnston, Tommy Curley, Tim Tom, Eugene "Buckskin" Charlie, Murray John, Pat McClary, Vern Bruhwiler, Ike Campbell and the like come to mind. Thanks to all of you and those not mentioned too.

Memories and Reflections on Program

"Ka Ka Wis has never been rigid" in its approach to alcoholism and other addictions. Instead, the Family Development Centre "takes a realistic and open approach", observed Ron Duffell, regional director of B.C. Alcohol and Drug Programs on Vancouver Island. Centre personnel see their work in its province-wide context. They recognize, he said, that Ka Ka Wis is one "complementary component in a series of services that work together in trying to overcome a very complex problem."

Each agency in this network contributes in an important way to the ongoing struggle against addiction. Many of the people involved work "behind the scenes", Mr. Duffell pointed out. They should not be overlooked in telling the story. Examples include the various care-givers who refer clients to Ka Ka Wis and provide before-and-after support in most native communities, ADP personnel who work out of Island headquarters, volunteers who give of their time and talents on the Board of Directors, and other partners in this continuous process.

* * * * *

As Ron Duffell observed, the Ka Ka Wis agenda has been changing and developing ever since programming began in 1974. This is evident when program schedules from 1975 to 1994 are examined.

This progressive development almost never happened, as a key player in this story confirmed during an interview.

If the B.C. Ministry of Health had accepted the recommendation of the Alcohol & Drug Program's first audit team to visit Ka Ka Wis, "it would have been shut down as far as the government was concerned". But a second and favourable assessment of the new Centre's work saved the day.

Walter Moy, program director of the ADP Outpatient Clinic in Burnaby, B.C., was a member of this second audit team nearly 20 years ago. He and Dr. Al Connolly assessed "the clinical impact" Ka Ka Wis was having on clients. The auditors were "greatly impressed by one of the most effective intergenerational counselling programs" they had witnessed up to that time, Mr. Moy recalled. Accordingly, the audit team recommended that the Centre should receive more funding from A & D Programs, which has been the main source of revenue ever since.

* * * * *

Some further reflections on program from members of both cultures in the Ka Ka Wis partnership:

- Dr. Evelyn W. Pinkerton, UBC Social Scientist, noted: "Ka Ka Wis grew up as a local response to the needs of west coast people." She believes that is one major reason the Centre works well. Its program is widely "perceived as a reflection of the people's culture," she said during an interview.

  "Local people made this grassroots effort work instead of choosing a highly funded model from California", or some other expensive import, she commented. Because Ka Ka Wis is a local enterprise "the people know its history, or do by the time they leave as clients. The island location is another important factor." Together, all these elements "make a huge difference" in terms of effective treatment.

- Kelly John, now of Gold River, was one of the authors of "The Kyuquot Proposal". In 1974 the proposal became the reality known as the Family Development Centre. Twenty years later, he was asked how he viewed the Ka Ka Wis program.

  "I think there's more awareness now that we need to do more ourselves rather than be so dependent on the program," he replied. "So we're planning to hold more workshops on healing." At the same time Kelly John reported that his two sessions as a Ka Ka Wis client had helped him deal with alcoholism. "Actually, I'm celebrating my eleventh or twelfth sobriety birthday."

- Howard Tom, Tla O Qui Aht band manager, welcomed news that a native woman elder had worked with Centre staff at a recent Ka Ka Wis counselling session. He had heard that Elder Columba Frank "had a lot to give to the young people who were there. They gained a lot of strength from having her there." Howard Tom welcomed this further sign that "the whole program is taking in more of our culture." He looked forward to more participation by aboriginal elders in the future.

- Elder Stanley Sam, Ahousat, spoke of healing from an aboriginal perspective. During an interview he first of all stressed: "We have our own culture. It's not a European culture. The Europeans have a written Bible, but ours comes through the plants here on earth, not through a book."

  He spoke of plants that "are our medicine to get rid of the evil spirit". Such plants have sacred names that cannot be spoken outside of cleansing ceremonies. Healings were not a form of magic, he stated. "You've got to know the prayer song for these things. You can't just sit there and let the plan work....It takes a plan and you have to work at it. And you've got to believe it, not just do it."

  Elder Sam said, "I quit alcohol on my own nine years ago". He expressed support for those clients who went to Ka Ka Wis. "We always have a celebration when the people come home from there. We give them a sober party and they explain how they feel about the place. Mostly they say that changing doesn't happen overnight. It takes awhile because alcoholism is a really big disease. It's some kind of evil spirit."

- Dr. Harvey Henderson, Tofino physician, described his change of mind about the main causes of alcoholism. "In occasional talks to clients at Ka Ka Wis I used to speak about genetic makeup and brain chemistry making natives very predisposed to alcohol. Then I met a counsellor here from Manitoba. He had been a skid-row drunk. He said alcohol use was a way of coping. It was a behavior people learned. It was not necessarily preprogrammed genetically but was more a product of a person's environment.

  "I've switched over to that side of the fence myself....But I'm also sure there is some chemical component as well."

Feelings

When she was program co-ordinator, Kathy Erickson/Seitcher often told new groups of client families what to expect during their stay at the Centre. Selected from a 1990 video recording, here is part of what she said:

"While you are at Ka Ka Wis a good part of the language we use will be about feelings. Sometimes that can be pretty scary, when we don't recognize what we're talking about. We're used to saying, 'I'm fine', 'I'm okay'. But inside there's all that garbage that no one's ever asked us about. And because nobody has ever asked us, we haven't even looked at it ourselves.... Whenever the pain does come to the surface, we choose to skirt the pain. It hurts. And we think it is our fault.

"Somehow, it's always our responsibility to feel good, to feel right, perfect. Nobody told us we would have all these feelings and that I would have to try to work it out so that I can be at peace. Even if I'm not happy sometimes, I know deep inside that it's okay to be sad, or to be angry sometimes. It's how I express that feeling that counts. Do I do harm to myself, harm my children, harm my spouse?

"Here at Ka Ka Wis we ask you a lot about feelings. Feelings you had as a child, and that maybe you've been carrying around for all this time. Maybe you're a grandma now, or a grandpa, and you're embarrassed to say you've had a feeling since you were 10 years old when someone really hurt you. 'I'm old now,' you say. 'I shouldn't have these feelings....

"Here at Ka Ka Wis we ask you to give yourself permission to have those feelings, to own them, to say 'I have these feelings and I'm still okay. I'm going to look at them. I'm going to ask help to deal with them. I'm going to learn how to be okay from the inside, from deep inside, to be peaceful.

"Addiction robs us of believing that it's okay to have feelings. Booze, drugs try to take away feelings so that I back out, make up, escape. When you choose to come here something deep inside you said you want to feel those feelings....We will come to a point where you can say, 'I can handle that. I know what that feeling is and I know I can handle it because I own it. It doesn't own me.'

"Then you can look at your children and say, 'It's okay not to be perfect. It's okay to have angry feelings. It's okay to be sad. It's okay to be happy. Whatever you're feeling, it's okay and we'll deal with it — together'."

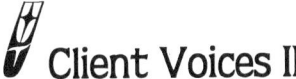 Client Voices II

Here's another representative selection of feelings and thoughts aboriginal clients shared during and after counselling sessions at the Family Development Centre. Their comments were chosen from the Centre newsletter, *Ka Ka Wis Star,* and from other records.

- A family man: " I could not accept the fact that I needed outside help until just before Christmas. That's when I decided to come to Ka Ka Wis. The six weeks I have spent here have been very rewarding. It has given me the basic understanding of my inner spiritual self.

  "I am grateful for being made aware of my inner feelings. Feelings I never knew had a 'light' and 'shadow' side. And that these were very important to each other, for they balance each other out. This has given me the foundation that I need to grow in spirit, and has renewed my faith in the Higher Power. Now I realize that I need to have faith in God so that I may nourish my spiritual inner self...."

- A young woman: "I learned a lot in our big circle. My husband and I were the youngest couple there. At first I felt like a child. Then I realized that no matter how young or old, we all had similar problems, one way or another."

- "I'm learning a lot about myself already. And I'm really enjoying myself here with my wife and son. And with my friends here too. I'm having a lot of fun playing volleyball with the guys and gals."

- A senior woman: "Understanding the family tree gives you a sense of identity and puts pride in you as a First Nations person, or whatever nationality you may be."

- A nine-year-old: " We had a sweat yesterday. There were 10 of us. My leg was healed by the sweat. It was fun. I jumped in the ocean. Then I washed up in the waterfall."
- "This place could work for anyone as long as you keep the circle strong....Accepting the truth was the hardest part. I made my decision. I choose to change, change for me and my family, change for the better. Kleco. Kleco."
- A client's poem, called "We Find Ourselves":

  "The men learn to become men once more.
  The women learn to love themselves.
  Our children learn to be children again.
  The ocean reveals life's mysteries.
  The rain washes clean every pain we have.
  The trees state that we will endure.
  To be one with life is to be secure."

- Why one youth felt right at home: "I really enjoy being here. Ka Ka Wis is just like home. Lots of quiet, beautiful and secluded. We are not overpopulated at home. We are a very small reserve. We don't have pollution, smog or all kinds of heavy machinery running all day long. I'm glad we don't have all that. But we do have lots of beautiful trees, birds and lots of water and a whole lot of space. No highways, buses, trains or pollution. Everything is natural."

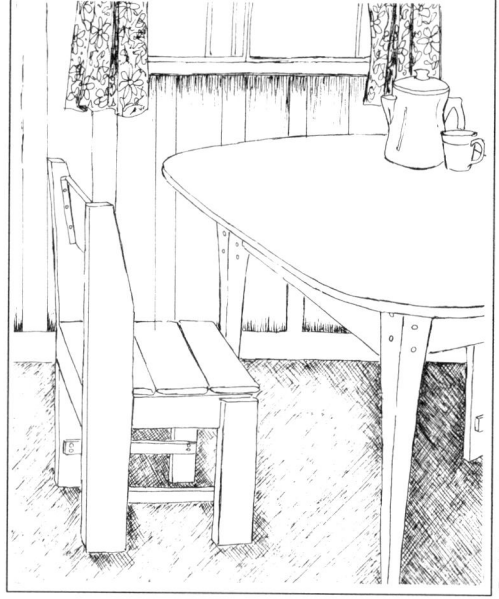

By Maureen Cato

- "We came in as strangers. Trying to remember names, who belonged to who. Can we really do it? Do we really want to? We've laughed, we've cried, we've opened our souls. We've told our pains and told our plans. We've bickered and complained, and we've shared our joys. We have been a great

Circle.... Thank you for putting up with my negativeness, my laughter and my sharing."
- One sibling to another: "I thank my sister for letting me learn how to get down from my ladder and get down to eye level and talk together."
- "I am so afraid to go home....I am scared I might get back to the disease. But, like they say, live one day at a time and think positive."
- "I realize the only person who can help me is me. I can get all the counselling in the world, but it's not going to do me any good unless I want it to."

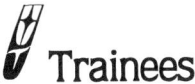
Trainees

By G.A.

Training at Ka Ka Wis brings to mind the five categories of life that we have to take into account in order to produce typical problem situations that will lend themselves to personal development when used as learning experiences for the trainee. The five categories are: self, family, leisure, community and job. Each trainee who is training here is either meeting "practicum requirements" or is training to fill a staff position. Trainees are required to participate in a full sessional program in order to experience and deal with ("problem solve") any personal issues they may have in their lives. Examples:

Self: Low personal self-esteem. Unable to communicate with others, trust in others. Fear of others dominating them. Fear of loud, angry people. Some come here with the gift of speaking, listening, singing, etc., and recognize that each ability is one they share with others.

Family: They learn to communicate with family, play with their children, take care of spouse's and children's feelings. They learn discipline procedures that work and don't work today. They learn helpful information they can share with their children about sex. They learn how to fight fairly and take "time outs".

Leisure: The program addresses many areas of leisure time one may have with oneself and with the whole family. Hiking, swimming, colouring with your kids, mask-making, trust walks, writing and relaxing. These are just a few examples that a trainee experiences.

Community: The trainee gets to participate in a new community that will learn to share, care and love one another throughout the program. "I make a difference." No one part of the Circle is greater than another.

Job: Sharing ideas they once kept to themselves. Developing their own personal skills. Trusting others and being honest with themselves. Learning to give feedback as information given with care and concern.

This is only the beginning. After fulfilling the program a new challenge presents itself when the trainee begins to work with the people in the program. The trainee develops his or her own style of working — "not the Ka Ka Wis style". The context of the program will always support itself. Then it is time to be consistent and practise, practise and practise the newfound skills that have led to a better and healthier family life. - G.A.

Smudgings and Sweats

After breakfast in their individual units, client families meet at the Social Centre. There they form a Circle. In the centre scented smoke is rising from a large sea shell of burning sage and cedar — sage from the B. C. Interior and cedar from the west coast.

Adults, youth, children and Centre staff come forward to whoever is conducting the ceremony. With a gentle upward motion of hands, each person "washes" in the scented smoke by wafting it about the face and head, arms and shoulders. Some pray in silence as they do so. Then a group prayer is offered — an invocation to the Creator, usually followed by the "Our Father".

This symbolic rite, which begins each weekday program at Ka Ka Wis, is called "smudging". It is one of the principal spiritual practices at the Centre. The other is "the sweat", described below. Both are optional, not imposed.

Ever since it began as a "Christian core community" in 1973, program and ceremonies have evolved at Ka Ka Wis. But the Centre has remained "a prayerful place". Trusting belief in the Higher Power — however that Presence is experienced and named — characterizes Ka Ka Wis.

"Spirituality and cultural emphasis are really important in our program," Carol Sadler wrote when describing the Learning Centre curriculum. And speaking of the program for adults and youth, Pat Koreski stressed the important role of rituals such as smudging.

"Smudging is just one of the ways humankind tries to reach out and communicate with God, using natural elements, whether it's smoke, fire or water," he said. "Holy water and the rosary are examples in the Catholic tradition." Whatever the spiritual heritage, the point is that "you use something tangible in trying to get in touch with your spiritual roots. I guess you could say all rituals are pathways to your inner self."

Smudging symbolizes an inner cleansing of body, mind and spirit. The practice originated many centuries ago among Canadian and American aboriginals east of the Pacific Coast. It is similar in intent and appearance to the ancient Jewish and Christian use of incense during religious ceremonies. Smudging also somewhat resembles some traditional rites followed in other ancient cultures.

Smudging is not an indigenous practice among the Nuu-chah-nulth peoples. Instead, each west coast native family traditionally has had its own private rituals, which cannot be shared. Ka Ka Wis honours this privacy. But so as to demonstrate respect for native spirituality, the Centre introduced the smudging rite followed by many First Nations peoples elsewhere.

A former client and staff member, J.C. Lucas, is credited with bringing both smudging and the sweat-lodge ritual to Ka Ka Wis. For centuries this purification rite has been used by many North American tribes. Thanks in good part to what he experienced in the sweat lodge at the Round Lake treatment centre, J.C. Lucas has sobriety today.

The Ka Ka Wis sweat lodge is located in a forested area near the main buildings. The darkened structure is heated to a sauna-like temperature. Those who enter the lodge for a period of prayerful reflection experience "a return to our mother womb". Like smudging, the sweat experience induces "a cleansing of body, mind and spirit," states a Ka Ka Wis program manual. "It requires an act of humility to sit in a fetal position, admitting powerlessness before our Maker. Disclosing our difficulties, sharing our problems with other people and in prayer asking for the needs of our inner self."

Pat Koreski stressed: "My approach to rituals has always been very cautious. We want always to show respect. We'll not do anything we shouldn't, and we'll do properly what is acceptable. Over the 20 years these practices have evolved. But always we have tried to show a strong respect for both sides, Christian and native."

The interviewer recalled a conversation with a Northern Saskatchewan woman. Her ancestors were Wood Cree and French-Canadian. Every week she received Communion at her parish church and also "did a sweat". The two experiences re-enforced her gratitude that she was both "100% Indian and 100% Catholic", she declared.

This reminded Pat of a young woman he had met in a local "talking Circle". Speaking of her mixed heritage, she said she was "proud to be native and proud to be white". Pat congratulated her. "'You're a bridge,' I said."

This young woman personifies what Ka Ka Wis aspires to be — a life-giving bridge linking two cultures.

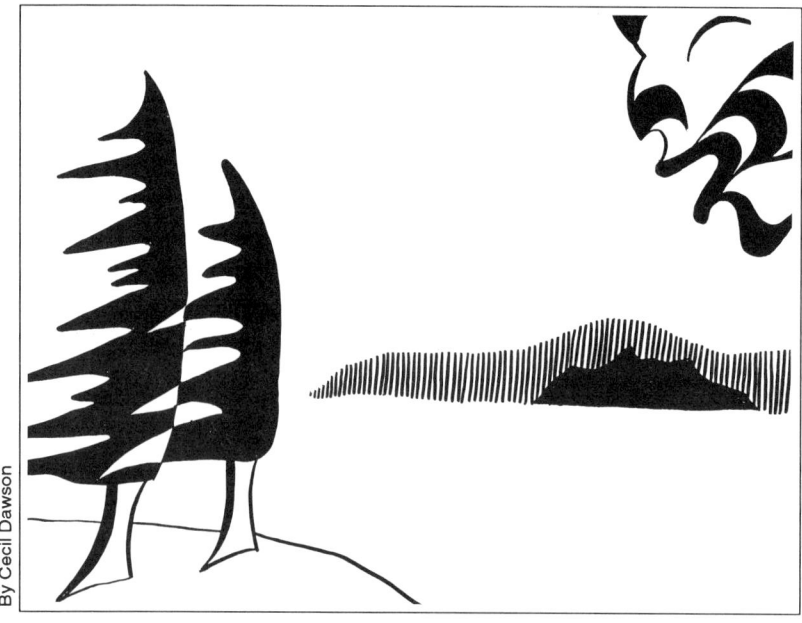

The Learning Centre

By Carol Sadler, Facilitator

When I became a part of Ka Ka Wis in 1980 the Learning Centre occupied three rooms on the second floor of the old residential school. During my first year there we were called Meares Elementary School, and were almost a separate entity from Ka Ka Wis. While parents were in session, the children attended school. In the evenings there were family games, birthday parties and some community suppers, but the children were not an integral part of the main program. It was a family centre only in that all family members were where separate parental sessions also took place.

School funding by the Department of Indian Affairs was given only for those who were "status Indians living on reserves". Since many of our larger client families lived off reserves, no funding was received for their children at Ka Ka Wis. The teacher had to be certified in B.C., but salary and resources were sadly deficient. Supplies left over from residential school days made it possible to continue, although students usually arrived without any. Library books, also left-overs, were old, with few pictures to capture the attention of reluctant readers.

The children worked on regular academic subjects, arts and crafts, and a small amount of addiction education. The only differences between this schooling and schools elsewhere were the geographic isolation and the fact that all school-aged children were in one classroom. Then, as now, working in the same class as brothers and sisters was a major distraction for students. The children worked on being aware of each other without interfering.

From the beginning, principals and staffs of Tofino and Ucluelet schools were supportive. Each session I was able to borrow books from Wickaninnish Elementary and Ucluelet Secondary School for the students who arrived without theirs.

Between 1982 and 1987 the school was staffed by Margaret Cantwell and Carol Proietti, Sisters of St. Ann, and by Marna Rogers, a Notre Dame

72 *Healing Journeys*

Sister (SND). The Sisters of St. Ann were extremely generous in providing both time and money.

The 1983 fire that consumed Christie Residential School buildings was a major setback for the Ka Ka Wis school program, as all material was lost and little of it was covered by insurance. Temporarily, the classroom was housed in a one-room trailer. Because funds were lacking, most of the replacement

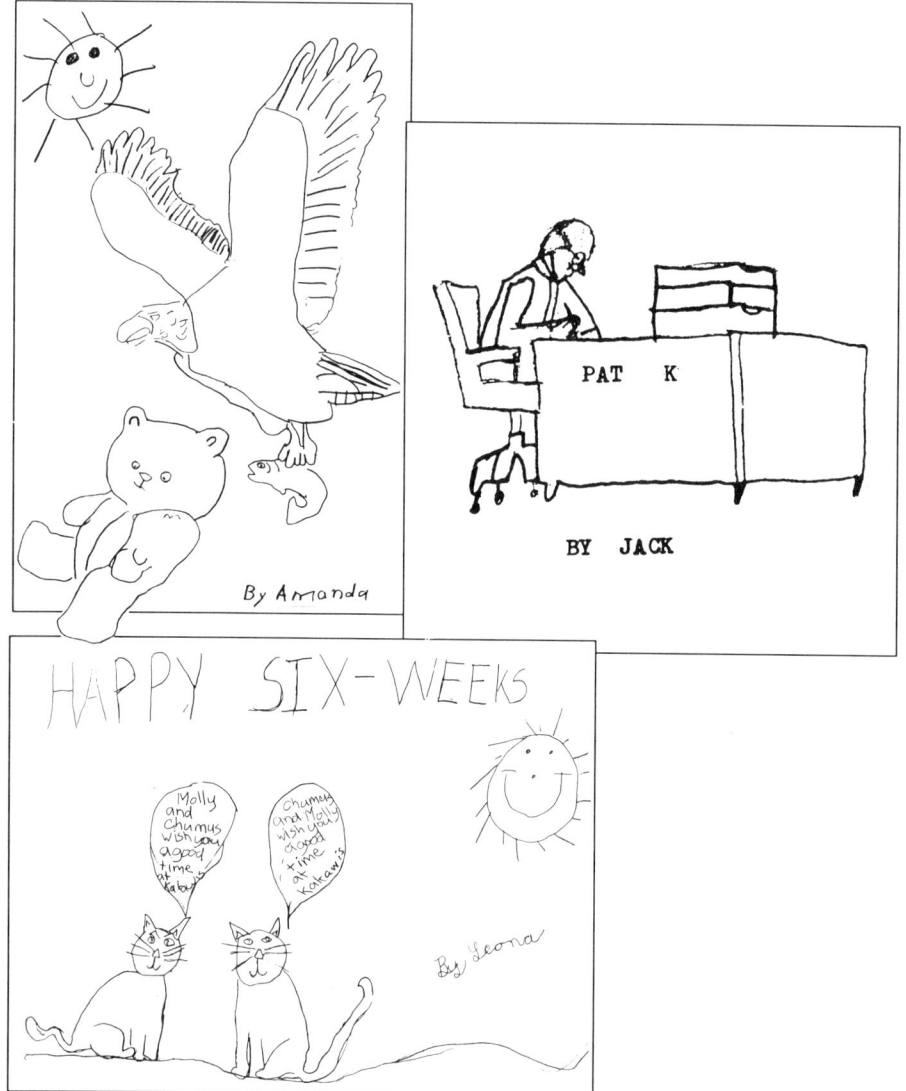

materials were even older and more worn than those replaced. The Sisters of St. Ann seemed to adopt the school as a priority and purchased new video equipment and new Montessori materials. Other supplies continued to be a problem as students still arrived with few, if any, materials.

At this time Margaret Cantwell was the teacher. She renamed the school The Learning Centre, and described her role as that of "facilitator". She began to take some aspects of the adult program into the classroom. The children learned some of the same things as their parents were learning, recognized and dealt with some of their own issues, and had their own Healing of Memories.

Although the children's issues were relayed to the adult counsellors, the children were rarely part of the adult circle. In the Learning Centre approximately 10% of the time was spent on "program-related material", and the remainder on academic work from their home school and on art.

We knew that to better serve the children, connection had to be made to the school system, with access to district resources. Thanks to the help of Norm Thiessen, Ka Ka Wis became a Short Term Provincial Resource Program under the direction of School District #70 in January 1987.

New resource materials and supplies were now purchased in advance. That September I returned to Ka Ka Wis as Learning Centre facilitator. After six years of teaching in the Alberni School District, I was aware of the resources available and the procedure to acquire them. The library was vastly expanded to include native stories and art books, as well as many other colourful texts. A series of games and other family-fun material were added to the library and were available to client families evenings and on weekends.

With the expanded budget, the Learning Centre soon entered the technological age with one Apple computer and printer. An electric synthesizer and a guitar were donated and used by students and adults alike. We looked forward to visits from Denny Grisdale, itinerant principal of Indian education, since he usually brought with him either a computer, a printer or news of one which was being supplied to the Learning Centre, which now houses five Apple computers, three printers, an IBM Compatible and an Amiga computer on which students create original art work and type the *Ka Ka Wis Star*. When Ka Ka

Wis purchased a new copier, the previous one was moved to the Learning Centre, much to the delight of staff and students.

The Learning Centre had doubled in size, new cabinets had been installed, and furniture acquired. All this became necessary when the number of students and the amount of equipment both increased.

The addition of a Cultural Resource Person to the Learning Centre team was another significant development. Once a visiting delegation arrived at the Learning Centre. Denny Grisdale, Rod Burke, the Tofino school principal, an official from the Ministry of Education, and Pat Koreski came in. They found me wrapped around a student to keep him from harming himself and others in his rage, with other students standing around almost itching to get involved in the ruckus. Pat said, "Maybe we have come at a bad time." Seeing that things were under control, the delegation stepped back outside to let things cool off somewhat. My first thought was, "Oh no! Now I'm done for!" But quite the reverse was true. Approval for a second worker in the Learning centre was soon received. Since then, a native person skilled in aboriginal culture has worked alongside me, beginning with Florence Frank, followed by Lewis George and then Viola Sparvie.

Another significant change began to happen when it was decided that parents and children should be brought together for aided discussion of certain issues. When children first arrive at Ka Ka Wis they are well grounded in the family rule of "Don't tell anyone our business or our family secrets!" They soon learn that they can trust the school staff, and through the use of carefully chosen stories, videos and activities, individual students learn they are not alone in what they experience.

Once one student has personally identified with feelings or actions of one story-book hero, and is able to speak of the similarity with his or her own life, choruses of "Me too!" are soon heard. These comments are punctuated with admonitions from older siblings: "Don't tell everything!", and "Mom (or Dad) will be mad that you said that!" Or there will be arguments about the truth of various statements and replies that "You know it's true but you just don't want to say so."

While confidentiality is necessary, many of the topics the children talk about need to be shared with the parents. Such issues are first discussed in the Learning Centre because the children will state their true experiences, feelings and fears once they feel comfortable with the facilitators. Whenever subjects discussed are intended to be shared with parents, the children are informed before they speak.

When the children's comments are shared with the adult Circle, the children themselves are present. The parents are encouraged to give their children verbal permission to say what they are thinking and feeling. Parents also are encouraged to share their own reactions with the Circle of families present. Each Circle member gains strength from the other, and the children gain trust and confidence in their parents.

Parents and children who attend session together are bound to be in a more positive position to support and understand each other back home. Family fun activities such as community suppers, scavenger hunts, Himwitsa (story telling), making masks, making pottery, silly games of Hokey Pokey and Alice the Camel, and serious games of basketball and volleyball, are some of the activities families choose to continue at home.

Another major difference between the Learning Centre and most schools is the important position of culture, spirituality and ritual. Every school day at Ka Ka Wis begins with smudging, prayer, hugs and "The Walk for Sobriety". The role of the cultural resource person is a demanding one since it entails bringing native culture into the classroom in a natural way, using it as a teaching tool and a source of pride, while also fulfilling the responsibilities of a teacher's aide.

Reactions of children in the program are reported elsewhere in this book. One of the strongest statements indicating that some measure of success is being achieved came from a 15-year-old boy six months after leaving Ka Ka Wis. When he saw me again in his home school he came up to me with his arms reaching out for the expected hug. He said, "You know, since I left Ka Ka Wis, you are the first adult who has looked me in the eye. Why is everyone so afraid to look you in the eye?... Before I came to Ka Ka Wis I was getting E's and F's. Now I'm getting A's and B's. It's all to do with being here in school every day. It's okay!"

A Postscript

"I was very impressed," said Ron Erickson, supervisor for School District 70, in summing up his visits to the Learning Centre. His office administers provincial funding in an area that extends from Port Alberni to Bamfield and includes Ucluelet and Tofino.

He conferred with both Carol Sadler and Pat Koreski on each visit. "I think the students gain a great deal being at Ka Ka Wis with their families, while not missing out on educational opportunities," he commented. "Probably they even gain by working in a small group with a teacher like Carol. There's a kind of family feeling with children of all ages working together. And the resources available are just excellent."

Recently appointed to his post, Mr. Erickson said he already has had school principals visit the Learning Centre when pupils from their local schools were at Ka Ka Wis. He planned to have room teachers visit "so they also get a feel for the whole program and how it involves all family members."

More Reasons to Celebrate

"There's lots to celebrate!" This enthusiastic comment by Joe Tom, Ka Ka Wis co-ordinator of community services, was echoed by dozens of others during 1993-94 interviews. A sampling of these mostly "upbeat" reactions:

- A 1950's pupil at Christie Residential School, later an adult client, and now a senior staff member, Joe Tom cited some of his reasons for celebrating. Two of them: "I celebrate our cultural differences. Ka Ka Wis is a place where the cultures come together and every one of us is the richer for it.... I also celebrate that many clients discover that life is worth living while they're here. Every day without drinking is a celebration for them."

- Peter Greig, Tofino accountant, part-time ambulance driver and Board member, said: " I'm impressed by what people of both cultures bring to Ka Ka Wis. Native people have a lot of fine characteristics that often seem to be lacking in non-natives. Once clients overcome alcoholism and related problems, they really are wonderfully vibrant people."

He described the Centre staff as "special people". As for the director, "Pat has almost a reverence for the place. It's a mission for him."

- "I see Ka Ka Wis as a very sacred place, "Sr. Carol Proietti, SSA, stated when describing her teaching years at the Learning Centre in 1984-87. "While there I came to know myself at a deeper level. Pat Koreski challenged me, challenged all of us, to achieve things I never thought I could do or we could do. I gained something immeasurable there."

Thanks to the appreciation of aboriginal cultures she gained at the Centre, Carol said she has since become an active supporter of native causes in the northeast U.S.

- Chief Francis Frank of the Tla O Qui Aht First Nation tribes (TFN) said the Centre has good reason to celebrate because it is much more than a drying-out treatment facility. "There has been the typical stereotype of Ka Ka Wis that it is just an alcohol and drug treatment centre. We've had a big struggle to get our people to see that it's a Family Development Centre that deals with a wide range of questions." Chief Frank said the Centre is doing the job it was designed to do. But its contribution to the struggle against addiction cannot succeed without more follow-up support by TFN and other native communities.

- "I celebrate the Ka Ka Wis I knew as the place where every individual discovered that precious person that each one had been carrying around inside for years," said Sr. Patricia Shreenan, SSA. "In journeying with many people there I did a lot of self-discovering myself.

"I also celebrate that you could enjoy the solitude there. Even though there were always lots of people about, you never lost the sense of solitude. At the same time I celebrate the way people cared for one another. Individuals and the whole community experienced healing together. The two were integrated."

- George Atleo, now associate co-ordinator, expressed hope that the 1994 anniversary celebrations would draw on the traditions of both cultures. "I'd like to see all the people who ever went through the program come back for the celebrations....I'd like to see a plaque with all the names on it, including those of staff members who have been here."

  He pictured a diversified and colourful event. "I can't see a lot of people just getting up to make speeches. Instead I see them involved in different ways." A healing ceremony, a scavenger hunt, a mountain hike up Lone Cone, and a salmon barbecue were among the possibilities he favoured.

- " I celebrate what I do here," Sherry Merk said with a smile. Her work in handling intake records and helping co-ordinate the outreach program to reserve communities keeps her in close touch with all phases of the Ka Ka Wis effort.

  "In some small way I'm helping people who have suffered a lot make a better life for themselves. I see such a contrast in people's faces when they arrive and then when they leave. At first you see scared faces, sad faces, people looking down. But by the last week you hear laughter and joking. You see tears and you see family members relating to one another with a lot of strength."

  Sherry also celebrates "as a woman because my work challenges my intelligence as well as my heart. I could make more money elsewhere. But if the choice is between money and happiness, I choose happiness," the single mother said.

- The Ka Ka Wis vision and program "celebrates the capacity we all have to change those things in our lives which limit our growth as human beings," wrote Marna Rogers, SND. She hoped the Centre "will share its experience with others....To this day Ka Ka Wis is the only program I know that brings the entire family into the experience in a holistic way."

- Carol Sadler estimated that more than 700 native children of client families had attended the Learning Centre during the previous five years. Whenever the Learning Centre facilitator visited native schools on the reserves she heard mostly positive feedback. "The kids who have been here are eager to tell me about the things that have changed since they were here".

- "I still have native kids call me," reported Gael Duchene, who helped redesign the Ka Ka Wis Youth Program in 1986-88. "One girl was seven when I first knew her and now she's 14 or 15. A couple more keep in touch by mail. That just points out how special Ka Ka Wis is." Gael celebrates this continuing connection with former client youth and hopes some day, when her child is older, that she may return to teach at the Centre.

- After several difficult months as the new program co-ordinator at Ka Ka Wis, David Zyrd experienced a breakthrough in what he was trying to do as a professionally trained counsellor. He and a once hostile client reached a friendly meeting of minds during one session.

  "This has given me new heart, new insights and new inspiration," David said. Now he has personal motivation to celebrate what the Family Development Centre stands for. "One of the central reasons for Ka Ka Wis is to model working relationships and fellowship between natives and whites. Now our counselling supports and encourages traditional native culture as a healing strength because of its spiritual values."

- The fact Ka Ka Wis is on an island is itself cause for celebration, Elaine Greig, Centre bookkeeper, said. "What a wonderful thing it is that there is such a place on a beautiful island away from stores, cars and other escape routes." Elaine cannot imagine Ka Ka Wis working as well anywhere else.

- Ray Seitcher, former Centre counsellor, celebrated the fact that two distinct cultures — aboriginal and "white" — work as partners. The best traditions of both cultures "teach respect for other people" and the Centre is living proof of that respect.

- "Absolutely! There should be a celebration!" declared Joe Leins, for several years regional director of the B.C. Alcohol & Drug Programs on Vancouver Island. The founders "had a vision and they put flesh on it," he observed in recalling the struggles of the pioneer staff. "It's a very spiritual place as well. And you could say Ka Ka Wis is helping aboriginal families regain their pride. I think the Centre is providing that kind of bridging in a very exciting way."

- Pat Koreski summed up: "If there is anything to celebrate, it's the healing. And what we're celebrating here is healing in brokenness. To me that is the number one thing we are celebrating. We cannot project for sure what is going to happen. But as Patricia Shreenan used to say, 'If we close tomorrow, we still have a lot to celebrate.'"

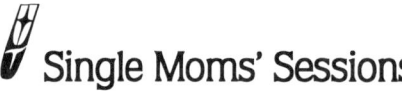

Single Moms' Sessions

By Sherry Merk, Intake and Community Services Assistant

When I took over intake duties at Ka Ka Wis, I soon noticed how many client applications came from single mothers. At that time we did accept single mothers into regular session, but required them to find a supportive adult to accompany them.

Often it was hard for these women applicants to find someone willing to go through the program with them. This support person had to be someone close enough to the client to provide the emotional support needed, and also share living quarters with a minimum of friction. Sometimes problems did develop between the client and her support person, leading to one or both leaving before the end of session, or at the very least, interfering with the client's focussing on the program.

The regular Ka Ka Wis program is very couples-oriented. Single mothers in the Circle often feel their lack of a partner very keenly when they see other clients working on their issues together as couples.

Being a single mother myself, I know that we have our own special issues and challenges, and a very different life situation to deal with. One difference often is having to cope with even more financial hardship than other client families experience. These and other special circumstances that single moms contend with could not always be addressed thoroughly in regular sessions geared mainly to the two-parent family.

When the Centre had accumulated a rather large number of single moms' applications, it was decided to try having a whole session of single mothers only, using all available units at the time. We would accommodate 11 or 12 single-mother families rather than the usual eight families. When word got out, we very quickly had an overflow of applications. All units were filled and there was a standby list.

The care workers who refer clients to Ka Ka Wis are very positive and enthusiastic about the results of these sessions. We continue to receive a flood of single-mother applications. We held the second single-moms' session in the summer of 1993 and once again had an overflow of standbys on the waiting list. So many, in fact, that we planned a third session for February 1994 rather than wait for summer. The February overflow would form the base for the next such session.

Counsellors note a dramatic difference in these sessions. Since all the women are in a similar situation, they connect very easily with each other. In the regular Circle counsellors sometimes find that women whose partners are present will be afraid to speak up and say how things really are for them, for fear of hurting or angering their spouse. There is no such hesitancy with the single moms! Every session they are open and verbal and very able to express their issues in Circle, right from the beginning. Staff also note the strength and humour evident among the women.

We have found that the single mothers generally have received more pretreatment counselling than many of the two-parent families, and have already done much work on themselves. Most have already experienced verbalizing, and have been working on their issues before arrival. Once here, they are very ready to get to work and proceed further on their journey of recovery and discovery.

One of the issues addressed that generally does not come up in regular family sessions is the tendency in a single-parent home for a child to assume the role of the missing adult. Or the child takes on more responsibility than is appropriate for his or her age because of the family's situation. In this session especially, clients want the program to include more counselling of mothers and children together so as to deal with the particular problems that can arise in single-parent homes.

In general Ka Ka Wis staff agree that these sessions are very successful and that there is a demand for more of them. Personally, I relate very much to the single moms as I have lived through their special challenges and know how tough it can be, and also how rewarding. Some of us call these clients "Tough Marshmallows". We really enjoy their time with us!

The TFN Experiment: Three Views

1 – As described by the Director

In the spring of 1993 Ka Ka Wis received a letter from Chief Francis Frank and the Human Resources team of the Tla O Qui Aht First Nations (TFN), asking us to set aside one session just for TFN families. We happily agreed to do that, with the understanding that the session would be in partnership with the TFN Chief, Council and staff. This was agreed. We had a number of meetings with the Chief, some Council members and some staff. We set aside one session for TFN families, and also conducted a one-week team-building workshop for TFN Council and staff.

This six-week session was different from former ones in that four weeks were on site at Ka Ka Wis, while two weeks were held in the community and were open to all TFN residents. We did this because we feel very strongly that it is the Chief, Council and community members who either support the family in their recovery effort or actually weaken the chances of recovery for them. There is no magic at Ka Ka Wis; it's not a "fix-it" program. What is done here is only a part of the larger picture and process of healing.

First there was preparation of families by visits from two of our staff to most of the homes at Opitsat and Esowista. Unfortunately, only five families and one individual attended this special session on site. But another 20 to 25 individuals attended some or all of the sessions in the community for the last two weeks. Due to land negotiations the Chief and some of the Council members were unable to attend the one week team-building session, but most of the staff attended.

There was a send-off feast in the community for the families that came to Ka Ka Wis. The Blue Bead ceremony, which is normally held at Ka Ka Wis,

The Evolving Program   **83**

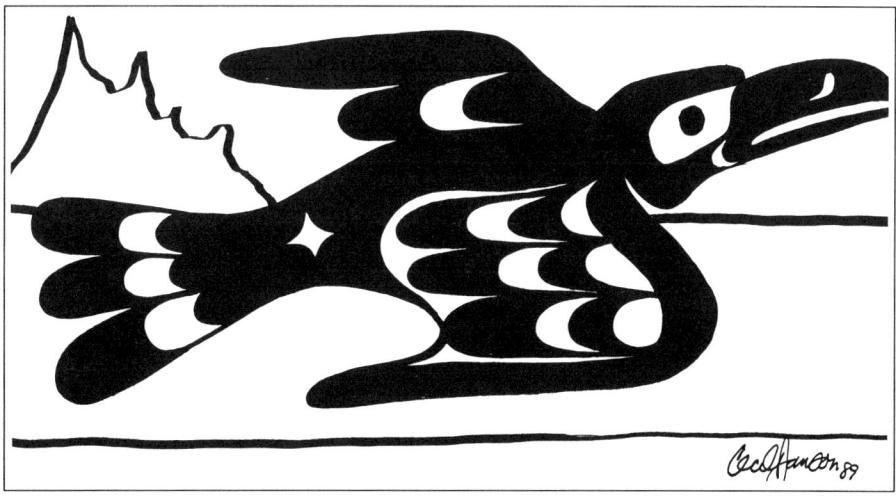

was held in the community. Also, three issues of a special newsletter were sent to every home in Opitsat and Esowista, informing all about what was happening.

The goal of the whole project was to make it a joint effort by the community and Ka Ka Wis, so as to bring about family and community healing and growth for the Tla O Qui Aht peoples.

The project was successful as a partnership and did bring about some healing. How much still has to be determined. The main interfering factors were apathy, denial and hopelessness on the part of some tribal members, and the extreme overload all leaders presently carry because of land and resource negotiations and self-government issues.

The concept of the TFN experience is a sound one, and Ka Ka Wis is open to attempting similar projects with other tribal groups.

2 – Two Native Views

During an interview early in 1994 Chief Francis Frank referred to the 1993 project organized jointly by the Centre and the TFN Council and staff. "Ka Ka Wis did their job," he said. "They helped the families get back on their feet during the six-week period. But some failures came once they left the safety net of Ka Ka Wis."

This showed, Chief Frank acknowledged, that the Tla O Qui Aht Council and care workers need to provide "more resources in the event that others get into the same difficulties."

When interviewed, Howard Tom, TFN band manager, also commented on the 1993 experiment. He referred to the Family Development Centre's handy location for most coastal tribes. This proximity contributed to the six-week session jointly organized by Ka Ka Wis and the TFN community. He felt it had "worked out pretty well".

Later Pat Koreski had facilitated a successful workshop for TFN employees, Howard Tom pointed out. "Our staff is similar to others in sometimes having tensions and not always working together. After the workshop with Pat everybody felt better. He is used to working closely with native people."

Other Centres

Ka Ka Wis is no longer the only residential family centre in Canada or British Columbia. In this province the Nenqayni Treatment Centre in Williams Lake now takes native families for residential treatment. Ka Ka Wis also has shared information and experiences with the Wah-Pox Detox Centre at Bear Lake, Alberta. This centre also takes families for residential treatment.

Spokespersons for both centres spoke positively about Ka Ka Wis when they were interviewed. David Ross, executive director of Nenqayni, first visited Ka Ka Wis when the Williams Lake centre was reorganizing on a new site. "I reviewed the Ka Ka Wis program, looked at its format and how it runs, much of which we incorporated into our program. We got a lot of clues at Ka Ka Wis.

"One of the differences between us, I believe, is that we probably do more individual family therapy," Mr. Ross continued. "On three afternoons each week we counsel each family individually, including childen able to understand. Each family also spends some time at the education centre with the teacher and other students."

"I liked everything about it," said Angie Gervais in speaking of Ka Ka Wis. A native herself, she visited the Meares Island Centre as a family counsellor from the Wah-Pow DeTox facility in Alberta. Wah-Pow, which serves four families at each six week session, "is slowly incorporating some parts of the Ka Ka Wis program."

Commenting on these centre-to-centre exchanges, Pat Koreski said it should be noted that Ka Ka Wis also works on both a formal and informal basis with other residential treatment facilities in B.C., and especially with the agencies funded by the National Native Alcohol and Drug Addiction Program (NNADAP).

"I have belonged to the National Native Association of Treatment Directors for almost 10 years, and as well have attended many meetings with the B.C. native treatment directors," he reported. "Our staff have participated in joint training adventures with other B.C. native treatment staff. As well we quite often consult with one another on concerns of mutual interest.

"Ka Ka Wis is proud to be part of this group of dedicated agencies," Pat emphasized. "I am thankful to have peers to learn from, and with whom to share and celebrate."

"What's Your Success Rate?"

By P.K.

"What's your success rate?" is one of the questions most often asked of Ka Ka Wis. Because the Centre has not had a reliable and ongoing follow-up mechanism in place, this is a hard question to answer. However, there have been several attempts to answer it.

In 1980, 164 adult clients were surveyed by Pat Donovan, SSA. These statistics are not at hand. In 1983, just after the Christie fire, Patricia Shreenan spearheaded a survey: 147 adults and their children were interviewed. A summary of the information gathered shows that of 80 adult responses, 68 had maintained improved relationships in their families, and 12 had separated from their families. Of 86 adult responses to the question of sobriety, 65 indicated a positive change in their sobriety pattern, while 21 indicated no change.

(The 10-year survey report included this statement: "The purpose of this study is to put together information concerning the experiences of family members after completion of their treatment at Ka Ka Wis. This information will assist Ka Ka Wis staff in making more effective the services offered to families seeking treatment at our facilities. The study will provide the staff as well with evidence of the durability of change which occurs in a person's way of life while at Ka Ka Wis. Staff members will take advantage of the opportunity the study provides of making public relations contacts in each area where the study is pursued.")

In 1985 Drs. Evelyn Pinkerton and E.N. Anderson conducted a follow-up survey in conjunction with their overall review of the Ka Ka Wis experience. They interviewed at least one adult member each of 23 families who had attended Ka Ka Wis since the 1983 fire. (This involved about half the total number of families who had been clients in that period.) Of 40 individuals interviewed, 19 had stayed sober since leaving Ka Ka Wis, and one person did not have an abuse problem when he came to the Centre. Three had often drank and had experienced no improvement. Another 17 were not drinking at the time of the survey but had had relapses. One of the most important findings in this survey was the importance of proper detox ("drying out") time and stabilization time before entering Ka Ka Wis.

In 1986-87 an audit team from the Alcohol and Drug Programs, B.C. Ministry of Health, did a review. They did not conduct a follow-up survey, but stressed the importance of that component, and recommended that this be done.

In 1989 a follow-up survey process was put in place by the Centre. Three simple questionnaires were used to determine the effectiveness of the program — one during the session, one after three months and one at six months. The most significant finding is that many clients still come to Ka Ka Wis without proper detox time or stabilization. Since the two mailings of questionnaires after the program are not followed up by further mail-outs and phone calls, the returns are too minimal to be statistically reliable. This procedure, however, is still in place.

In May of 1993 the Centre conducted a phone survey of all the past client families since January 1989. Either a family member or a referral person was contacted. The main purpose was to determine the sobriety rate. Of these 254 clients, 112 reported they had maintained complete sobriety, 58 had not, and 32 we could not determine. The significant finding in this survey was that female clients had a higher success rate in our program than males.

All these surveys indicate that Ka Ka Wis does have an impact in lessening substance abuse with families. The need for a more structured and reliable follow-up plan is there, but doing it would mean more resources or a shifting of resources.

Two Other Views of "Success"

Joe Leins, for a number of years the Vancouver Island director of B.C.'s Alcohol & Drug Programs, was asked about the Ka Ka Wis "success rate".

His reply: "I don't get any clear picture of the success rate regarding sustained sobriety....From the available data, it looks on average like at least a 35% success rate. I think it's probably better than that but you can't really prove this. It also depends, of course, on the length of time period you measure....

"We need very clear assessment standards at the front end of all such programs in the province. Then we will be able to say what the 'success rate' is in each particular period."

When interviewed by phone, Dr. E.N. Anderson of the University of California recalled his working visit to Ka Ka Wis in 1985 and answered the "success-rate" question this way: "Fifty per cent sobriety after one year is about what Ka Ka Wis seems to get...This is an extremely high rate for one year after an average treatment program."

But the anthropologist stressed that this rate is "not out of line" with reported success rates for other North American programs that also include "native components", as the Ka Ka Wis program does. Nowadays this blending of cultural elements in programs is pretty well "standard practice" in Canadian,

American and Australian centres that serve aboriginal clients. The presence of native values and practices in programs contributes to commendable rates of sustained sobriety afterwards.

There are two theories as to why these programs work so well, Dr. Anderson continued. "Most would cautiously say that it's because treatment is more culturally appropriate for the native clients. But some others, including myself, stick our necks out to say that the traditional beliefs and healing methods of many native cultures have a great deal to teach everybody everywhere when it comes to treating alcohol and drug abuse, and other conditions that have a strong psychological component."

Dr. Anderson remarked that the dominant North American culture "tends to put down so-called primitive medicine because it doesn't cure infectious diseases. But it never really pretended to do so. It deals with psychological conditions."

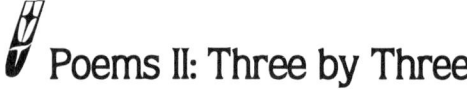 Poems II: Three by Three

"Little Brother, Little Brother"

A teen-age sister mourns a younger brother. She shares her grief and resolution with readers of the *Ka Ka Wis Star*
My brother was crying with no tears.
I didn't know he was hurt and had a lot of fears.
He hid his fears with laughter and jokes.
I miss him. So do a lot of folks.
He killed himself, which makes me mad.
I said to myself, "Bro, you got the family sad."
He lost his reason for living. He gave up.
I still love him but I can't forgive him.
Little brother, little brother,
We were just starting to be close.
Little brother, little brother:
I know I got to let you go.
You'll always be alive in my heart.

I won't let our memories together go apart.
I know you're dead.
I got to put my life ahead.

Alcohol

A client at one Single Moms' Session composed this poem.

Little girls of years ago,
Witnesses, victims of tragedy,
Playing roles much older than ourselves,
Not by choice but by alcohol.
Pain and tears all stuffed inside,
The years slip by, we smile, we laugh.
A scream inside is never heard,
Not by choice but by alcohol.
Young girls entering womanhood,
Knowing only what we've seen and heard,
An unhealthy cycle consumes our being,
Not by choice but by alcohol.
Our children are our precious gifts.
We care for them as best we can,
Distracted by illness, our energy's wasted,
Not by choice but by alcohol.
Our spirit's broken, yet we rise.
We start to see clearly, we recognize
the beautiful person within,
the peace and serenity each day can bring.
So, to all my friends as we go our own way,
the tools we can practise with each new day.
We have been shown an alternative way to live,
Not just for you but for your kids.
I say "Kleco" from a place within
where anger and pain used to be.
We have shared so much, I will miss you all!
I won't let you forget me,
I'll give you a call —
by choice, without alcohol.

Ka Ka Wis By the Sea

Composed by a male client, who also provided a drawing.

*Ka Ka Wis, the beautiful place by the sea,
It will always be here for you and me.*

*It's a place to learn a new lifestyle
in what seems to be a little while.*

*It's a place of letting go,
a place to come and grow.*

*When it comes time to leave,
there's a part of us that wants to grieve.*

*The staff will give us encouragement
to go and share our personal development.*

*Thank God for this beautiful Ka Ka Wis
— the place everyone will grow to miss.*

– A.J.A.

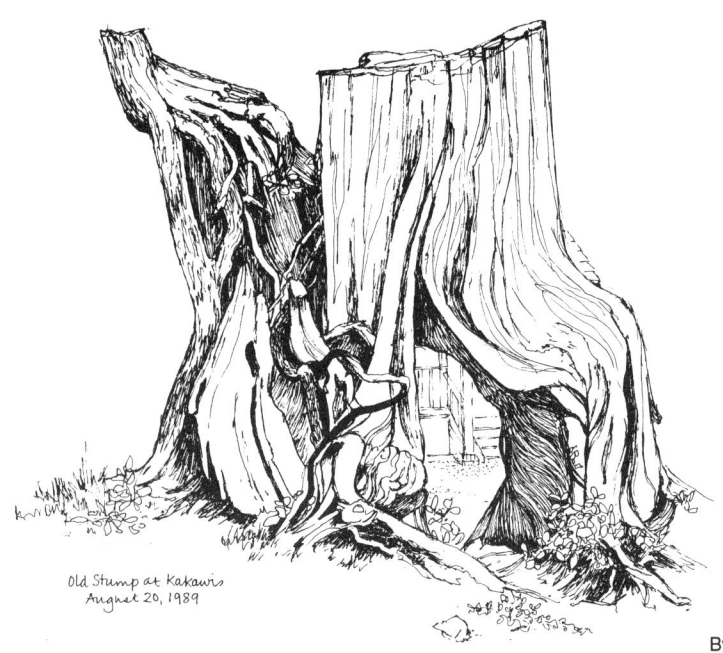

By Maureen Cato

Healing – Experienced and Shared

Where's Healing?

By P.K.

Where is justice, where is freedom, where is healing? At the heart of pain, in the centre of the cycle of violence are these questions. And the way they are answered will ultimately determine whether this passing on of hurts from one generation to another, in families and out, will continue or finally be stopped.

I believe each of us has to look deep within and search out and accept as ours the evil destructive forces that lie within. This is not an easy task and it requires supreme honesty. It requires help from above. It is the crucifixion side of spirituality.

If these evil forces have already been unleashed by me on others, then the question that haunts me is, "Am I worthless, have I any good at all, do I deserve any happiness?" Fear becomes my companion and doubt tempts me to give up and kill myself physically, emotionally or spiritually. If my spirit dies, I am free to lash out and live my evil by spreading more and more abuse, whether verbal, physical or sexual.

If these evil tendencies have been kept in check in me and buried Oh! so deep, then pride can be my companion and denial can tempt me to reach false conclusions and make wrong judgments. It is easier for me to cast blame and demand retribution than it is for those who must live with guilt and regrets.

If I am a victim of these destructive acts — rape, beatings, verbal assaults, abandonment, it is so hard for me to bear the pain permeating my whole self that anger and hate become my companions and vengeance tempts me. Punishment lies to me and tells me "getting even" can heal, can take away my pain. My pain that feels so unbearable.

If I am both victim and offender in this cycle, I become confused. I fluctuate. Fear and anger and hate and confusion become my companions. At times I can make excuses and be tempted to minimize my guilt and responsibility. And at other times I can hate myself so much that death looks soothing. The forces within me are so strong it often becomes unbearable. Whether I am a victim of these destructive forces or the causes of them or both, addiction can help me cope. Addiction to alcohol or other drugs helps me forget the fear and hate and pain I feel inside. Helps me mask my own responsibility or mask my shame, suffering and feeling of worthlessness.

How do I live with all this and make any sense out of it? How do I reach my potential as a special person? Or for me is peace, is serenity only an illusion, a false dream? Have I been created only to suffer? Is there simply just good and evil, and was I unfortunate enough to have been born on the wrong side, or fortunate enough to have been born on the right side?

These are serious questions and their answers have very serious consequences. As a Centre, Ka Ka Wis deals with this reality daily and finding the answers to these questions is central to our work.

Someone Special

One of the clients told the story. When she was preparing to come to Ka Ka Wis, a friend told her that she would meet someone there who was very special. She would know when this happened. As the weeks went by, she kept looking for this special someone. Near the end she found this person and she was very surprised. It was herself.

"The Circle is Sacred"

"A circle has no beginning and no ending. It is complete and the space contained within the circle is shared space. Participants in the Daycare Centre, the Learning Centre and the Adults Program meet each other and staff members by forming a Circle. The use of the Circle at Ka Ka Wis has been described as 'sacred', 'precious' and 'spiritual'.

"Traditionally, the native Indian has taken his problem to a Circle consisting of a concerned person who was party to his particular problem and the elders. There are certain rules of conduct in the Circle. Interruptions, advice-giving

94 *Healing Journeys*

and criticism were not acceptable. Listening, sharing individual experiences, story-telling and looking at alternatives to solve problems were acceptable. An individual thus supported was free to stop the process at any time.

"In the program at Ka Ka Wis the members of the Circle learn to listen, to trust, to share, to respect, to risk and to care. All members of the Circle have equal status. The use of the Circle is central to the program. Concerns of clients and staff have been resolved successfully through the Circle. The preferred way of learning by native Indians is experiential. The Circle is experiential."

— **Ann Tasko, researcher/ writer,** *The Tasko Report,* **1987, p. 53.**

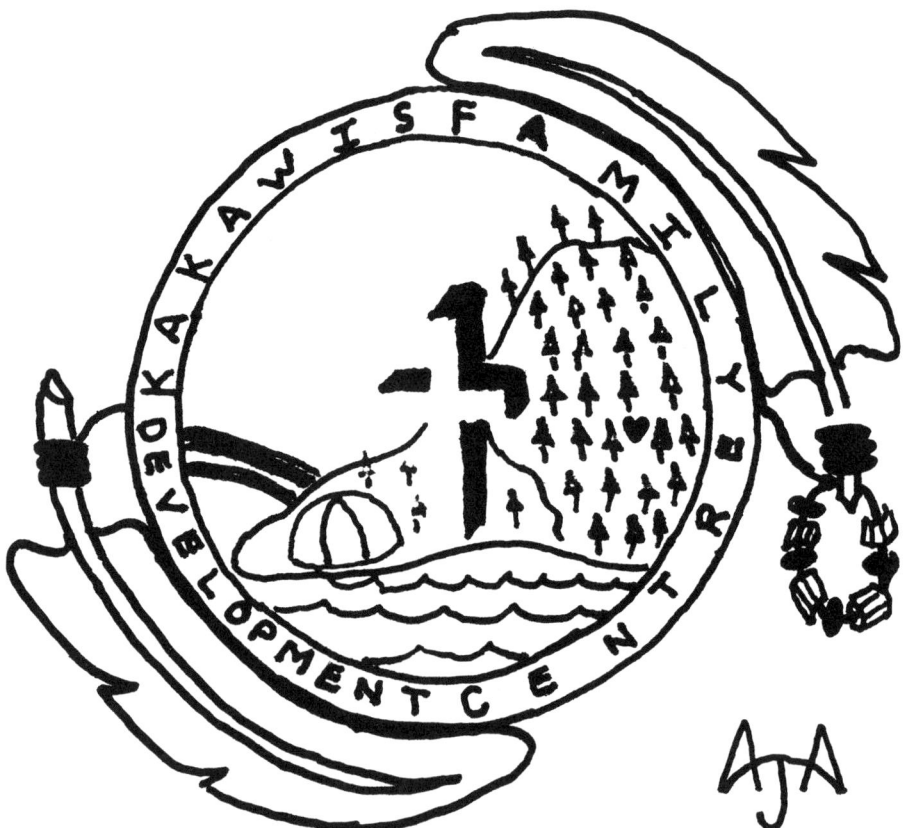

My Journey so Far: Joe's Story

Hi. My name is Joe. I would like to share the story of how I felt before I went on a healing journey. Some very personal parts will be left out. I will say things that may offend some poeple. Or this may open their eyes to recognize what we need to do on a journey of healing, to have a better life.

I was born in 1944. It's a beautiful thing to have been born. But as time went on I was called a "bastard". For many years I never really knew why, but that's what I was called. I was also called a "spoiled brat" who "got everything you want". Things like this affected my life at a tender age.

When I was five and a half I was sent to residential school. I came to Ka Ka Wis, which was called Christie School then. I was excited and yet scared. I remember being called "a lefty", which was taboo. I should use my right hand, not my left. So I got the nickname "Lefty". I learned I had a temper. I learned to fight and hit back because I was called names.

My mother died at a young age. I happened to be in school when she died. I cried. I wished I was there. I thought mom wouldn't have died if I had been there. I can't remember my age then. I don't seem to want to remember.

Back at school again and lonely. I spent time going into the woods and dreaming of being home. At school we were taught that we had to learn English. We had to learn the ways of the white man. This was the only way we could amount to anything in this world. I was never very good at spelling so I would get whacked on the head. "Spell it right!" If I still didn't spell it right, I got whacked again. So I became hard, I became cold.

I couldn't do a lot of the things I wanted to do because rheumatic fever had weakened my heart. I didn't really understand this. In sports I tried, and again was ridiculed for not being good enough.

In religion I learned that I had to be a good Catholic. I must do this and not do that. When at home I went to Sunday school, but I got ridiculed for going because I was a Catholic. When I went back to the Catholic church, I was told it was a sin to go the Protestant church. A lot of this talk came from my own people. I don't think they realized how much it hurt. What kept me going was my dad, and my mom before she died. They said there is only one God, one Great Spirit. That kept me going.

The church says you should never think or talk about things like sex, and you never ask questions about sex. "It's bad. It's no good". At the same time you hear the opposite from older brothers. "This is what you've got to do. This is how you do it. You got to do it this way. If you want to be a man, you've got to do it now." If you didn't do what you were told, things were done to you. Things that are unmentionable here. These were meant to frighten me and I learned well. And there were hurt feelings.

At school I would get strapped. I would just stand there and stare at them, not showing any pain. So I would get more. In my mind I was saying, "I'm not going to show you I'm gonna cry. No way!" Being told that you're nothing, that you will never amount to anything, because I stood up for rules and commitments we had made to have better sportsmanship. All the names I was called. "You're a lefty, you're a devil, you're not human, you're different." I would fight back. I was told to control my temper but wasn't told how to do that.

I left Christie without graduating. I understood it was because some of us were radicals. Because we stood up to our teacher, our supervisor. At the same time we were told, "You have to get an education to be someone". I had to learn the European style.

My dad wasn't doing too well fishing. Things weren't as good as they probably could have been even though he worked hard. He worked hard so I could go to high school. Once more I was away for 10 months from my father -- a man I appreciated very much and love very dearly. It was very difficult being far away in the B.C. Interior and not allowed to go home. On my first day in high school one of my native brothers from the Interior said, "You fish head, you better watch out what you do here or we'll box your ears off. " I said, "Come and try it. Take your best shot. " I was learning to be tough. I joined the young soldiers/cadets. Again I had difficulty because of my heart. But I insisted, got checked out and was finally accepted. That was the first time I felt I had accomplished something. I felt accepted.

Later, as a young married man, I worked hard to prove myself but ran into obstacles again. Lke hearing, "You can't make over $100. You have no business being a fisherman. You'll never be a good fisherman. You'll never get rich." I did a bit of logging also. At 23 I went to work in the boom in Ucluelet. Doing good, working hard, proving I'm worth something, that I'm a capable person.

We lived out at Long Beach. Nobody else was there at the time. It was nine miles into Tofino. To get our groceries we had to walk or get a ride. A young man in Tofino wanted to sell his car for $800. I had $400 so he says, "Why don't you go to the bank and borrow the other $400?" I phoned the bank and they said to come in tomorrow. So the next day I was there and said I wanted to borrow some money. But the bank man said, "Sorry, I can't." "Why not?" I asked. He replied, "We're not allowed to lend to natives." Then you shop in a store and you can hear a non-native lady yelling at her kids, "Quit running around like a wild Indian." Again, thrown in my face.

Even with our own people, when playing sports, working, not going to drink with others. Being called "goodie goodie" and told "You think you're too good for us". So I started drinking too, just to please. Only to find that I couldn't handle it . All my anger would come out when I was drunk, and it didn't take much for that to happen. By now my feelings were, "Why bother? What's the use?" But then I'd say, "I'll show them. I'll show them I'm a man."

All those years of being criticized, as if there was no right way. If I was right, it was wrong. And if I was wrong, it was really wrong. This went on in my relationships. I didn't seem to be good enough to do things right. At one point I walked the beach and tried to figure what was going on. I stood at the water's edge and said, "What is going on with me? How come I am the way I am? How come I can't do anything right? How come I can't please anybody? I can't seem to make people happy?" As I stood there I thought, "God, how easy it would be to run into that water and end it all. Then I wouldn't have to worry." But when I heard myself think that, I went away from the beach saying, "No way am I going to give them the satisfaction of doing that!"

For about four years I kept saying, "Gee, I've got to do something. There must be something better. Why do I feel that I have to keep proving myself?" By this time I had forgotten everything that was beautiful in my life. I had forgotten I had family. I had lowered my self-esteem so much that I didn't really give a damn. Yet I needed attention.

Finally, I said, "Oh what the hell, I'll go to Ka Ka Wis." I came to the Centre with the lady I lived with at the time. What happened in our group during the six-week session stays there. But I can tell you that there was a lot of awakening, a lot of pain. A lot of what was happening to me, I denied. I said, "No way. That never happened. I don't need this. I don't need anyone to tell me how to live." At the same time I would reach out to them, I would listen, and they kept telling me, "You're the only one who can do it, but we'll walk with you." But I always said, "I heard that story before. Nobody gives a hoot. Society doesn't care. We are told to be little white natives, but we are not accepted."

After a year I went to the Round Lake Centre reluctantly because different things had happened in my life which had been dealt with in a Circle -- and that's where it stays, in a sacred Circle. I went to Round Lake and learned more about my life. I learned who I was then and why I was becoming the way I was. Again, this is not said to hurt anyone in my family or anyone else out there.

This is where I learned that I must reach inside of me, reach that "Little Joe" who long ago lost his mom. Who always asked for his mom when he was

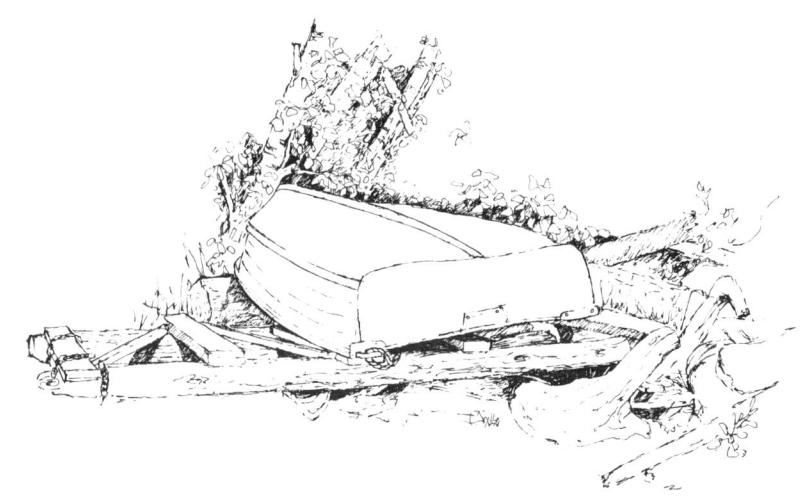

hurting. "Mom, I wish you were here. Mom, why did you leave? Why did you die? Is it my fault because I was at school?" I was always looking for blame for my mom dying. Not understanding why. Only to find out that I was angry with my mother for dying because she wasn't there through my teenage years and young adult life. She wasn't there to teach me.

But she did teach me about love and kindness. I know that now. With all the pain and hurting I couldn't see that for a long time. When I did accept my mother's death and grieved for her, I let her go. Now I can talk to her. I can see the beauty she gave me. It's not shadowed any more by all the hurts, all the name calling and the other things I went through that made me feel like nothing. Back then I couldn't see the good people who were there in my life.

I thank the Great Spirit for the opportunity to walk the journey of healing. I know that the Spirit has walked with me. I know that he has walked with me, or she has walked with me. I am grateful to all my brothers and sisters who have walked with me in this journey, and how we have been able to help one another keep going. We are learning about the good life, learning about love, respect and kindness. And that is all we want to give. We are breaking the cycle!

The Blue Bead Ceremony

Every four- or six-week session at Ka Ka Wis reaches a dramatic climax when the Blue Bead ceremony occurs near the end of the counselling period. "Graduating" clients exchange the beads as they make a hopeful vow to trade in past drunkenness and domestic chaos for future sobriety and family peace.

"Trade" and "hope" are the key words. Both words came to mind when Gerry Guillet, then priest director at the Centre, found some trading beads on abandoned reserve land elsewhere on Meares Island.

It was July, 1981. He, the Centre staff — including natives Louie Frank and J.C. Lucas — were busy making plans for a three-day celebration of sobriety on the long August weekend. The program was to include a sunrise ceremony on two successive mornings, a potlatch and other highlights.

The beads Gerry discovered reminded him that the treatment centre at Round Lake gave glass marbles to clients when they completed the program there. The marbles reminded former clients that those who went back to drinking would "lose your marbles".

On the August weekend at Ka Ka Wis, the Oblate priest reasoned, why not use blue beads in a similar way to honour all those who had completed the Centre program since 1974 and had continued along the road to recovery?

Gerry Guillet described his inspiration in a 1983 edition of *Kerygma*, a pastoral periodical published in Ottawa.

An excerpt:

"The bead I had found was saying many things to me, but basically two. First, it is a trading bead used years ago.... to 'rip off' the Indian...a hurting memory of the past. However, the symbolism is still valid: trade...to exchange one thing for another. This ....could today remind them of what they had just traded off. In their search for sobriety...they had traded off drunkenness for sobriety, insanity for sanity, a worthless life for a priceless life....

"The second symbolic meaning of the bead is linked closely to the first meaning. It can remind them....(that) there is hope! There is new life! There is a new dawning. There is a new Sunrise!" (Pp. 39-40)

The first Blue Bead Ceremony followed that August. About 150 beads were presented by Centre staff to all former clients who had returned to Ka Ka Wis for the celebrations. Since then hundreds of clients have exchanged beads with one another, and many parents have given beads to their children as pledges to trade in the old destructive way of life for healthful and peaceful living.

The public ceremony takes place at the Social Centre or in the gymnasium. Since the

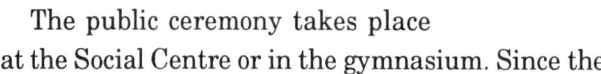

by Maureen Cato

spring of 1988 the Dance Curtain has provided a powerful background to the living drama that family members, relatives, friends, visitors and staff witness. Prayers, songs, hymns, drumming and dancing contribute to the emotional impact.

Marnie Andersen, west coast author now living in Sidney, B.C., shared impressions of the bead ceremony she observed in February 1987. Part of what she wrote:

> *"The bead signified the trading of one's old life for a new and different one. Each person was to fashion a necklace or bracelet, to be exchanged with another, a fellow journeyer down this, the new road. Faces were strained now, voices lowered. It was much like preparing for a final examination in feeling, honesty and love. All were aware, however, that it was not a 'final', but a 'beginning'. What followed next was one of the most beautiful communions of the human spirit I had ever been privileged to witness....*
>
> *"Pat spoke briefly of 'washing the mirrors of our inner beings with the healing water of tears' and told us, men and women, not to be ashamed to experience these emotions."*

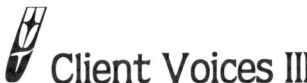
Client Voices III

A concluding selection of reflections, hopes and concerns voiced by native clients, first shared in the pages of the *Ka Ka Wis Star* or other Centre records:

- "This is my life I am talking about and which I want to heal....I think God has given me a purpose for taking this session."
- "At Ka Ka Wis I began to walk, journeying through my life.

    My secure and happy days with grandparents, Mom and Dad, and at the same time feeling angry. I am beginning to recognize feelings and to accept and share my innermost feelings.

    "There are ways of life I treasure......I have a deep respect for my forefathers. I have a feeling of reawakening of this sacred part of me, and I no longer feel lonely and alone....I feel I'm beginning to connect with my grandfathers on the Four Directions, and on the importance of the four seasons to put my life back in balance."

- "At Ka Ka Wis I learned how to communicate with my children, how to play with them. After I shared my story about my life with my boys, they began to understand why I was the way I was — drinking and trying to commit suicide. After I shared with them I felt so much better about myself. I learned to forgive others and most of all forgave myself."

- A boy writes: "I wish I could live here forever but I have to go back to the city so I can go to school and meet my friends. I like the beach at Ka Ka Wis, I like to look at the mountains. It is quiet here. A lot of air. Nicer people here than in the city. I hope to come back another time."

- A man speaks: "Coming over here on a Sunday, two days late....there was a lot of mixed feelings. A lot of it was being ashamed to be here, ashamed that I needed somebody's help. Over the course of the years I had never ever reached out. I had never asked anybody to give me a hand in anything."

- A woman's voice: "It was just my mate that had the problem. But in the sessions here I found out I had down deep hidden feelings, and why I was the way I was from that secret that was hidden from when I was five years old. I wanted to throw my life away. I thought I was worthless. I thank my mate for having a problem, for helping me find my problem."

- "Usually every day I go and walk on the beach, or go to the dock and sit there and think, especially when it is a nice day like today.... That really helps me to let something out."

- "I've seen some positive changes in some families at Ka Ka Wis. I feel very good to see the young ones during smudging. Four boys have gone through the sweats with me."

- "Somehow I couldn't help but wake up at six this morning. If I slept any longer, I might waste a precious moment at Ka Ka Wis. Thank you, God, for bringing me here. I am now stronger to become the child you have in mind for me to be."

- "What the Blue Bead will mean to me, upon leaving Ka Ka Wis...I will chip away the anger, resentment, blaming, self pity and all other things that made me very sick in alcoholism. I will become a different form of person in my new achieved sobriety."
- "There were plenty of reasons why I wanted to quit boozing. But not knowing it was FOR MYSELF as well as for the children....I feel very proud of what I learned at Ka Ka Wis."
- Two months after returning home, one client reports: "I'm not afraid to admit about being at Ka Ka Wis. So far I'm still SOBER — living one day at a time. Two months is not very long but it's a beginning."

More Recent Memories

Some memories of the Family Development Centre's second decade, shared during 1993-94 interviews and selected from the *Ka Ka Wis Star*:

- Dr. Evelyn Pinkerton has "many lasting memories" of the several weeks she spent at Ka Ka Wis in 1985 as visiting observer. One of her most vivid memories is of a group counselling session led by Patricia Shreenan, SSA. From Dr. Pinkerton's enthusiastic account:

    "Several couples and older children worked together for several hours. They did a number of exercises that were extremely provocative and moving. Sometimes there were role plays as clients played out a family history. The person whose history is being played out chooses others to play the family roles. The story is told and the people playing the roles change body postures. Then at certain moments the action stops and people are asked to talk about how they feel.

    "Then there would be a break. After that each person goes into the Circle and tells what it was like to play a role. This helps the person whose life is being played out to understand what people in that position were experiencing.

    "For example, I was asked to play the mother of one client. This person's mother had had children when very young, and the person had felt abandoned by her mother....I was able to talk about how it felt to have this load of children....I told her I just loved and adored her but that it was hard for me to focus on that sometimes because my husband had left me with this big family. The client understood from this that some of her mother's behavior, which she as a little child had interpreted as pushing her away, happened because of what her mother had to go through. Then the client was able to remember some signs of her mother's love.

"What astounded me about this family drama was how easily people could identify with the roles they played. How powerfully these situational dramas spoke for themselves! How universal the situations are!....The dramas were centre-pieces for people to express emotions and deal with them.

"I think one reason this exercise was so appropriate for the Nuu-chah-nulth people is that it is mostly non-verbal....It is well known in group therapy that for people of European ancestry vocalization and rationalization sometimes get in the way of expressing feelings.

"I'll never forget the powerful experience of that day. That was by far the most powerful therapy I had ever experienced. I was in tears many times."

- "I have never looked back since that day," Mabel James said, recalling the helping hand she had received from another native woman on arrival at Ka Ka Wis as a client in 1982. Mabel, now a counsellor, said that because of a dream she was "really scared" about crossing a small bridge on the road to the Centre.

  Margaret Andrew, the Ka Ka Wis resident then accompanying the newcomer, reassured Mabel. "Then Margaret said, 'Are you ready to cross now?' She said it in such a gentle way. I said, 'Yes, let's go.' She reached over and squeezed my hand and away we went.... Now when new clients come, I always remember that and put out my hand to them like Margaret did to me."

Healing – Experienced and Shared **105**

- The three men who have served as directors at Ka Ka Wis since 1973 have been described "as different as oil and water". How do they remember one another on the job?

  "Jim was really good as an administrator and I was the dreamer type who came up with new ideas," Gerry Guillet said when describing his working relationship with fellow Oblate, Jim MacDonell.

  Asked his memories, Jim chuckled, then replied, "Gerry and I were a good combination, I suppose, but it was frustrating sometimes."

  Both former directors commended their lay successor, Pat Koreski. Jim described Pat as "a combination of us both — a dreamer who is a good administrator at the same time." Gerry said, "But for Pat we wouldn't have survived."

  Pat Koreski emphasized the distinctive gifts and dedication of both predecessors. "They were very different, yet they complemented one another well. Jim was thoroughly organized and a hard worker.... Gerry was the charismatic one. He had a wonderful way of making people feel welcome."

- A native parent, writing in the *Ka Ka Wis Star*: "When I was 14 I left home on my own. My Dad kept drinking. He sank lower and lower. My brothers grew up. They drank. I drank. I never stopped crying. Then I had children of my own. I hurt them the same way my Dad hurt me. But at Ka Ka Wis I learned all the hurt I carried had to be set free. Now it's over and gone. I'm myself. I'm me. I made mistakes. And my children understand."

- "At Ka Ka Wis I saw 'miracles'," Margaret Cantwell, SSA, said. "People came in so bent, so broken. They were revived during the program....They literally straightened up and looked so much healthier." What she witnessed reminded her "how Jesus healed the woman who had been bent over for many years with ailments."

- "Nobody could go to Ka Ka Wis and not be touched by it," Dr.E.N. Anderson stated when the California anthropologist described his working visit to the Centre in 1985. "My most wonderful memory was being with the people. Everybody was working so hard to make themselves better persons. Clients worked with staff and staff worked with clients. It was just a very warm, very human experience.

"I took a lot of solitary walks and meditated on what I was experiencing and learning. That has stayed with me, and certainly has turned my life around in a number of ways."

- Marna Rogers, SND, who in 1985-86 taught younger children at the Learning Centre, wrote: "I continue to draw on those learning times with the children, whose courage, resiliency, honesty and simplicity I value so much. Even now these children often come to mind. I wonder how they are and hope that healing time continues to nourish their families."

- "The most vivid memory is the openness of the children once they have been at Ka Ka Wis long enough to trust you," Carol Sadler said. The Learning Centre facilitator was asked how this trusting atmosphere was fostered. Her answer: "There's lots of calmness. We talk about respect. We stress the positive, not the negative. And there are lots of hugs — safe hugs. They know that what we're doing is not going to turn violent, is not going to be abusive."

- First in the Seventies and later in the Eighties Bob and Maureen Cato worked at Ka Ka Wis — initially as volunteers and then as staff members. Both have warm memories of some working colleagues..

"Brother Reg O'Brien is the most memorable person in the whole place," Bob Cato declared. "There's got to be at least half a book written about him alone. Get some insights on Reg and his life story from other people there because you won't get anything out of him about himself....There isn't a native person he doesn't know on the west coast, going back three or four generations."

Maureen Cato spoke with equal warmth about Jack Ryan, staff counsellor and recovering alcoholic who later died in his native Ireland. Pointing out that she was "not at all religious", Maureen said, "Father Jack was so down to earth. He helped us when our daughter-in-law was dying of cancer. He was a tower of strength. He never mentioned religion. I admired him all the more for that."

- "Healing" and "feeling at home" are some of the first words that come to mind when Patricia Shreenan, SSA, remembers her years at Ka Ka Wis in 1981-85. "In my experience, Ka Ka Wis was a place of healing in every possible way. It was a place where people could be themselves, could feel at home. There was never any need for roles."

- Caroline Linitski, experienced volunteer counsellor at Ka Ka Wis for short periods in the Nineties, observed: "I was impressed most by the honesty and humility of the native people. They really wanted to change, to take responsible control of their lives.....They want to regain the wholeness of family life and break the culture of home abuse."

- "Coming here was like a feast in heaven," wrote a client in the *Ka Ka Wis Star*. "I had been to similar feasts many times before as I attempted recovery but I didn't concentrate on the food that was good for me."

  At Ka Ka Wis a different menu was served. "First there was the dish of admitting that I had a problem. Then acceptance.... Then the main course came along, and that was 'letting go'.... I had to let go the ugly taste of sexual abuse, the physical abuse, the emotional abuse. By eating this main course I had to let go of all the garbage in my system....

  "The dessert consisted of platters of hope, trust, loving, sharing..... I really stuffed myself.... What a meal! Thank you Ka Ka Wis. Thank you for the people who passed the food to me but didn't force me to eat. Thank you for choosing the other guests to share the meal with me. Coming there was like a feast in heaven."

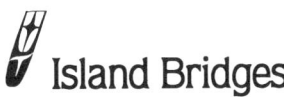
Island Bridges

By Munro Mabey, Director, ADAPT Society, Nanaimo

An Island Bridges committee was formed in October 1987 to create an opportunity for native and non-native alcohol and drug workers on Vancouver Island — who are funded by the National Native Alcohol Drug Program (NNADAP), the B.C. Alcohol & Drug Programs, and Friendship Centres —

to come together. The vision to come together to foster understanding, develop awareness and build positive relationships was clear. But we would have to wait for a clearer picture of how to realize these goals. Our first conference in June, 1988 at Ka Ka Wis would set the stage for what was to become a yearly journey in healing.

People from separate systems and separate cultures came together to share, to listen to one another, to laugh, to cry, and to care for one another. A new and expanded community was created — a giant step taken toward building a support and healing network for workers in the alcohol and drug field. The evaluations of those who attended the first conference reflect the power of learning from one another:

- ...a healing experience....I returned with an increased positive outlook on life generally, and clearer in my goal of better health for the (whole) client.
- It reminded me of the great cultural benefits of knowing our local heritage. I loved reconnecting with native people, there was so much caring, understanding and sharing.
- Meeting people who share a spirit of co-operation and a vision for health strongly told me that we are not alone.
- Gave us hope things really can change.
- Touched by a spirituality that I haven't experienced before.
- Gratitude for gathering together in healing.

The first conference created the venue for later gatherings. By offering an opportunity to share our experiences and ways of healing with one another, Island Bridges has become a place to come together as healers, to refresh ourselves spiritually, physically, mentally and emotionally. From the sweat lodges, pipe ceremonies, message and grief work to the beautiful beaches and the spirit of caring that Ka Ka Wis exemplifies something beautiful happens each year at Island Bridges. As one of the participants poignantly said, "I was refreshed.... I saw things differently." And it continues to be so for those who follow.

Seeing things differently means different things for different people. For me it meant seeing the end of one search and the beginning or extension of another. The end of a search that began with my grandfathers and grandmothers and an extension of my own spiritual journey.

That journey has not been without difficulty or challenge. I knew many wounds had been inflicted on First Nations people by my race and so I was cautious at first about native people. I didn't fully understand what I was looking for, nor if I would be welcomed. Yet at a deeper level I sensed there was something about native people and culture that could help me. I was both afraid and drawn to that thought. I realize now that it was the rich spirituality of the native people and culture that I sensed and which attracted me.

My personal healing and training, to that point in my life, had been extensive, involving many counselling and group sessions, from Gestalt to Transactional Analysis and many others. I had grown immensely from those sessions but it was at my spiritual core that the call for healing was coming. The spiritual healing that my grandmothers and grandfathers had come to this land in search of, after four generations I had found. It was where it had always been, never lost, but in the culture and healing practices of the native people.

Through Island Bridges — "A network of healers joined by a common thread of Spirit" — I have been able to affirm my fundamental beliefs and dreams about the world as I would have it — a world where people of all races heal the wounds of the past. Where in the present there is a place at the inn, of honour and respect, for all people, races and cultures. All my Relations!

Concerns, Hopes and Celebrations

In 1994 celebrations and congratulations are in the spotlight. But off stage, deep concerns and anxious hopes persist. The unfinished war against booze, drugs and other addictions continues unabated in many households, at Ka Ka Wis and at similar centres. Always, it seems, hundreds of persons, dozens of families, are in need of a helping hand in their struggle.

Just how desperate situations can be is evident in the self-assessment reports that three applicants prepared when they enrolled for the Ka Ka Wis program.

- A woman in her thirties: "I lost my parents through alcohol and my grandparents. I have fun drinking, but when I get these blackouts I don't like it. I wake up somewhere and wonder how I got there."
- A 16-year-old client: "I would like to change from alcoholism and drugs and be myself. A more responsible person. Get rid of the hurts, anger, frustration, the shame, the guilt, my low self-esteem."
- An estranged husband: "I was no good to hold on to a wife. I'm an alcoholic and lost all my family to it....Alcohol is all we knew. We made it, sold it and drank it. I was co-dependent from day one....All that is left of my life is my son. I feel afraid to burden my son when he is just a child with his own troubles....Physically, I'm not all that well. Mentally I'm contemplating suicide a lot. I feel like a loser at the end of his rope. Spiritually I'm a mess."

* * * * *

Meanwhile, numerous former clients of Ka Ka Wis and similar programs celebrate their so-far successful efforts to stay sober and get on with life. Once desperate but now confidently hopeful, one such client celebrated by writing to the Centre newsletter:

"When I left Ka Ka Wis I had two goals: to get my own apartment and to go to school. I am now renting a nice condo. And I'm going to school!....It's a native school top to bottom and I love it. The course that keeps me going is native studies. I'm learning our history. Our teacher is basically showing us how to know who we are. I have gone through a lot of emotion in this course, but I have pride in myself and in my people that I never really thought about before....

"I live one day at a time and right now my only goal is to get my grade twelve equivalency. Next month will be my one year of sobriety! I have surrounded myself with people who help keep me on the straight and narrow path — mostly my family and my school, where my healing is ongoing."

* * * * *

Other hopes for the future and some concerns too were expressed by respondents during interviews in 1993-94. While joining in the celebration of the Centre's 20th anniversary year, many also had new goals to propose for Ka Ka Wis. Here are some of the comments heard.

- When he was native-resource specialist at Ka Ka Wis, Lewis George made sure beliefs and values of the coastal aboriginal culture were an important part of the Centre program. He would like to see more of this cultural emphasis. "A lot more healing needs to be done here and in the communities. The hurts aboriginal peoples experienced from Europeans have to be healed." For example, Lewis would like to see native elders sharing their wisdom on a regular basis with Centre staff and client families.

- "Yes, it's professional. They've done a wonderful job at Ka Ka Wis, but they could do still more," Joe Leins said when he was ADP regional director. He noted that the 1991 assessment of the Centre program carried out by Carol J. Savage provided "the documentation they need to move ahead on community outreach on the reserves, and it sounds like this is going well so far."

- Tommy Curley, former Board member: "One of the biggest things missing is enough follow-up after the program at Ka Ka Wis. The Centre is doing a good job…but when you get back out there where all the wild things happen, it's hard to stay on the right track. That's where the big problem is. We need more follow up out there."

- Carol Sadler agreed that Ka Ka Wis has "to encourage a better support system back home where clients live." She hoped more small support groups would be formed, composed of former clients. These would provide common forums where, without fear of outside gossip, former clients could discuss their successes and failures along the road to sobriety and family peace.

- Ray Seitcher, former Centre counsellor, voiced another concern: "When some people stop drinking they get into other addictions, such as bingo and other forms of gambling. A lot of our people are getting hooked."

Often unemployment is a major factor, he emphasized. "Most of us native people are not very good at promoting ourselves." What's the answer? "The answer is inside. We just need other people around us to believe in us so that we can believe more in ourselves." With more self-confidence, most aboriginals would make a better case for themselves when job hunting.

- "I used to wonder what would happen if Pat ever left, but that's not a concern any more," Tom Cavanaugh, OMI, said. "I see native staff there who want to carry on, realize they aren't ready to take it on right now, but also know they are going to be ready and will have the ability when the time comes."

- Counsellor George Atleo pictured Ka Ka Wis as a future resource centre — "one where we would be able to offer life-skill programs, job-readiness programs and educational programs". Then trainees could pass on what they had learned to native families when counselling them in their home communities.

- Caroline Linitski, former volunteer counsellor, advocated "more emphasis on better qualified personnel, whatever their cultural background." Qualifications for counselling positions should include "the ability to accept positive criticism and to be self-critical." She questioned hiring mostly former clients when recruiting personnel. In her opinion, this "is too blinkered an approach...and is too bound up with trying to heal the native culture." The real challenge, in Caroline's view, "is to extract what is best from both cultures."

- "I'd like to see more parenting skills taught for young moms," said Rose Tom, who cares for preschoolers at the Toddlers' Learning Centre. Many young parents "don't seem to know how to discipline their children so we have to try to teach them some rights and wrongs.... Some children will learn but some others just won't listen." Rose is prepared to attend a workshop in order to acquire more effective skills she can also pass on to young parents.

- David Zryd, program co-ordinator, also stressed life-skills. "Parents trying to gain sobriety need to develop skills so they can cope with the everyday stresses of life back home. If you can't cope with these stresses, you'll go back to drinking. If you can't work out problems peacefully as spouses, if you can't care for your children without beating them, all these difficulties will take you back to alcohol or drugs."

David also stressed that high unemployment, consequent idleness and boredom, plus welfare dependency were continuing sources of this family stress. "So I'd like to see us fit into the retraining and employment picture" more effectively.

- "The goal is to see that family healing happens as much as possible in the native communities, and that Ka Ka Wis in turn becomes a resource centre," Pat Koreski said in summarizing recommendations in the 1991 report, *Expanding the Ka Ka Wis Circle*. "It's our compass, The report points out the way we need to go.

"The less you intrude on clients' lives the better," he continued. "If people can get what they need in their home communities, they shouldn't come here. There is nothing magic about what we do here during four or six weeks. What the Centre does is give families a chance to slow down, assess where they're at, pick up one or two life skills and get headed in the right direction.

"After that there's still a lot of work to be done on the road to full recovery and wellness. Then it's up to them, the Creator and the people around them near home."

Pat looks forward to the day when the Centre staff become "trainers of people who will be effective supporters of native families in their own communities."

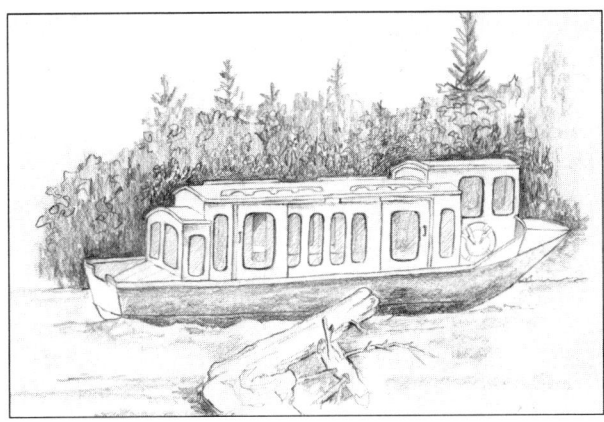

By Maureen Cato

Will the Bridge Hold?

By. G.M.

One often quoted description of the Ka Ka Wis partnership appeared in the 1987 *Tasko Report*, prepared by B.C. Alcohol & Drug Programs. It reads:

"The Ka Ka Wis program is providing a bridge for native people. The bridge provides a crossing from a place of cultural oppression, a place of perceived powerlessness, which is the legacy of the interface between Western society and the native culture in the last century, to a place of strength and freedom which permits choices to be made. Through this healing process the native Indian in today's society will be free to choose the best of both cultural heritages." (p. 74)

Since that interpretation was written, the pressures of several public issues have disturbed the foundations of the Ka Ka Wis bridge. Among the issues causing tremors: frustrated expectations of native self-government, prolonged negotiations on land claims, angry disputes over fishing rights in B.C., plus the marathon confrontation between environmental and logging interests along Vancouver Island's west coast. Add to these a now-settled 1991 land dispute and economic boycott in Tofino, plus the conviction voiced in some quarters that Ka Ka Wis should become a wholly aboriginal enterprise.

The 1991 program assessment, *Expanding the Ka Ka Wis Circle*, recommended better networking between the Centre and native communities, as well as improvements in program content. A follow-up report in June 1992, Exploring the Circle, summarized "feedback" received from some 40 sources, including leaders and staff of the Nuu-chah-nulth Tribal Council.. Among the feedback highlights:

"• Ka Ka Wis is perceived as a safe and healing place...;

- Partnership cannot exist without trust and understanding...;
- Outreach services must initially focus on networking;
- Ka Ka Wis must share with other resources how it uses cultural practices and spiritual teachings;

- Ka Ka Wis should focus healing for residential schooling on Christie School;
- Ka Ka Wis should tell its own story and celebrate and share its successes." (p. 2)

Sincere differences of opinion are heard on how best to strengthen the Centre program. Here is a sampling of views expressed when present and former board members and staff, plus other associates, were asked to comment on the partnership and its future prospects.

* * * * *

"I celebrate the fact that at Ka Ka Wis the two cultures are trying to work together," Pat Koreski said. Then he added: "But it has its tensions — there's no doubt about that. We are experiencing the winds of change.

"A bridge works because you have two steady pillars. But one of the pillars is not doing so well right now....We're under stress. I guess we'll have to live through it and perhaps changes will have to be made. Times are changing."

He recalled a comment made by a pioneer staff member and former program co-ordinator: "As Kathy Erickson used to say, Ka Ka Wis has always been a very fragile place.... We can't say it's going to last forever. It's a living organism. It's people. Our human brokenness is our weakness and also our strength."

* * * * *

Lewis George, native resource teacher on the Ka Ka Wis team until mid-1993, looks forward to the day when "all our people will stand up proudly". Traditional aboriginal teachings and rituals are major factors in bringing about this native revival. Lewis wants to see more of these traditions included in the Ka Ka Wis program.

The former school administrator at Ahousat, now a Tofino merchant, focused on these cultural values when he worked with client families. With Carol Sadler he taught children at the Learning Centre and also counselled parents in some adult sessions.

"How are the two cultures relating now at Ka Ka Wis?" he was asked. "Obviously there is a relationship but there has to be more awareness on both sides," Lewis replied. "Many just don't know, so there's a lot of ignorance that needs to be addressed....

"There are some things that you can't translate from one culture to the other. Our elders have been talking to us for thousands of years about these matters. So I think it's really important that we have elders here at Ka Ka Wis." (In an earlier discussion Lewis had named five elders — three men and two women —who he felt could share valuable learning with Centre staff and clients.)

"I really feel that in future Ka Ka Wis, sooner or later, has to go with our own people," he stated. Native personnel could "administer what happens here" and would be best able to address the issues that matter most to aboriginal families.

To describe the cultural revival he hopes for, Lewis told the story of a 75-year-old native woman who "got her youth back" at a Potlatch celebration. "This old lady was barely able to get around. But when she heard the singing and the drums at the Potlatch, she was totally revived. She was filled with new energy and soon was up dancing.

"That's what I want to see happening" in aboriginal communities, Lewis said in summing up. "And it's great to see that finally it is happening."

* * * * *

"If Ka Ka Wis were an all-native operation, my gut feeling is that it would lose some of its community support," said Don McGinnis, veteran board member. "I think we need the mix of native and white at Ka Ka Wis. For Tofino, Long Beach, Ahousat and Opitsat, that cultural mix keeps us in reality. All of us have to share this part of the world and make it work."

At present, Don McGinnis observed, there is a balance of native and non-native personnel, of recovered alcoholics and of those who never were addicted, on the Centre program and support staff. "This balance is important. In my opinion we should maintain this kind of balance." He also emphasized that "land claims and other public issues have no place on the Ka Ka Wis agenda". The Centre has more than enough to do in the family counselling field.

* * * * *

"I am more at home here at Ka Ka Wis than I ever was in my home town of Port Hardy," declared Mabel James. Why? Because "I feel the Centre program now is really living up to its name of family development" for native clients struggling to overcome addictions and repair home relationships.

"A lot of good changes have been made. Now the children are more involved in some adult sessions and the families are working harder at becoming a whole family unit. Also," Mabel continued, "I see things like sexual abuse, grief, losses and communication problems being faced up to and worked on. Now there are more counselling sessions with the whole family. I find it all really strong."

* * * * *

Volunteer counsellor Caroline Linitski, now retired in Raymond, Alberta, expressed concern about some developments she had observed at the Centre in 1993. "I became aware of an aggressive push to introduce more native culture into the program. Of course there are good things in the native culture and also less good things, just as there are in the white culture and all cultures."

The challenge, she said, "is to extract what is best from both cultures. The native counsellors owe it to the client families who come to the program not to give them the feeling, the conviction that they just have to go back to native ways with an uncritical attitude and then everything will be fine."

* * * * *

"Ka Ka Wis works okay for some clients," part-time maintenance helper Tommy Curley reflected. "But you can see that a lot of clients find it hard to talk to people of the white culture. They end up getting angry, but then after awhile you see attitudes change by the last few weeks." Speaking personally, he said, "It helps me just to watch the program helping other native people."

* * * * *

Dr. Harvey Henderson, Tofino physician, is enthusiastic about the cultural partnership at the Centre. "Ka Ka Wis is a very special place," he said and cited an example. One recent summer he and other medical practitioners who deal with alcohol and drug addictions met at the Centre. "Joe Tom led us through some of the native exercises," such as the smudging ceremony, the talking circle and the sweat lodge experience. "It was a very powerful experience for all of us", Harvey said.

"Exciting things are happening at the academic level as well as in people's daily lives," he pointed out. For example, "there's a whole new movement in family therapy coming out of Australia that deals with the oppression of aboriginal peoples and white colonialism."

* * * * *

"That's one of my goals — learning my culture," said Florence Frank, care-giver at the Toddlers' Centre. She had to give up speaking her mother tongue as a pupil at Christie Residential School in the 1950's-60's. "It's still really hard on me now because I'm still ashamed of my culture," she explained. "I can't even say a little word out loud, even though I can speak some" of the native language. She hopes that this will change as she learns more about her aboriginal roots.

* * * * *

"Probably the tensions between native people and white here are not any greater than the differences between loggers and environmentalists," said Vince La Plante, OMI, until recently Catholic pastor in the Tofino - Ucluelet area. He was asked what he had observed as a comparatively recent newcomer to the Island's west coast. Both areas of tension tended "to flare up" from time to time, he noted, and perhaps to a greater extent on the logging-preservation issue in the last year.

* * * * *

Joe Leins, former ADP regional director, stated: "For 20 years Ka Ka Wis has been one of the bridges for working together in a common cause — sharing knowledge and experiences, sharing cultures. I think Ka Ka Wis has provided that kind of bridging in an exciting way."

* * * * *

"The white society is just beginning to learn from us. So now each culture is respected and each culture shares with the other," said Joe Tom, Ka Ka Wis community-services co-ordinator.

Respect for native customs by the majority culture was a long time in coming, he noted. And in some quarters of Canadian society the prevalent attitude persisted that aboriginals were just "drunken Indians". But alcoholism "was never our custom before whites came," Joe pointed out. "Our bodies couldn't handle it when it came into our lives.

"And that's only one of the things that put us down. The reserve system meant nothing was really ours. This took away our pride, our self-esteem because we were treated as dependents."

The young-looking native grandfather declared: "Here at Ka Ka Wis I've learned how I want to be treated. You can't say to anyone, 'You're nothing.' Every person is beautiful, unique, separate."

Joe Tom spelled out the message Ka Ka Wis says by its actions: "Help one another to get back your life. Find self respect. Walk together. Share with one another.... Come and have a sweat with me. I'll not tell you what you should get out of it. You take from it whatever you need."

* * * * *

Carol J. Savage, who prepared the 1991 assessment of the Ka Ka Wis program, shared her "strongest feeling" about the Centre: "Ka Ka Wis for me is a place where peoples of two cultures come together to meet under a Higher Power. In the way that I understand spirituality, that is what is holy about Ka KaWis... It is one place where members of both cultures can become healthy."

* * * * *

"There is a strain on the bridge in some people's minds," acknowledged Ray Seitcher, former Ka Ka Wis counsellor. Asked how he would react if the Centre were staffed by aboriginal personnel only, Ray, himself a native, replied: " If that happened, some native politicians might take over and that would make it a whole different thing. I don't think we would be ready for that.

"That's me, although some younger people might welcome that kind of political interaction with a treatment centre," Ray added."But I could never see the two together."

But at their best he did see the two cultures sharing "respect for other people". At Ka Ka Wis, he stated, "the two traditions are together on that belief", even though mutual respect is not always practised.

* * * * *

"The Ka Ka Wis experience is happening at the same time as a bigger movement is occurring within the native culture," noted David Zryd, program co-ordinator. "The aboriginal culture is rediscovering itself. Native people are reclaiming their heritage. A lot of healing has to take place."

David feels the Family Development Centre is making a contribution to this healing process. "Ka Ka Wis is a light that helps some native people get back in touch with their culture and gain more self esteem." Speaking personally, he said this cultural revival had added an "unforeseen twist" to his job. "I came here wanting to help, but my help has not always been accepted." Why? Probably because he personified for some natives the white professional authority they no longer accept.

"It's a big challenge for me personally, but I'm more hopeful now than I was." Also, he said he was receiving more support and co-operation from clients, other staff members and from professional colleagues in Tofino and Victoria.

* * * * *

"It all depends on what you're referring to," answered Moses Martin, once a native member of the Ka Ka Wis Board, when asked how he felt about relations between the two cultures on the coast. "If it's about fish, there's a lot of bitterness between whites and natives. But on environmental issues, we have some common concerns."

Did he think, as some aboriginals do, that there should be more native personnel on the Ka Ka Wis staff? "I don't know if that would make a great deal of difference to me," Mr. Martin replied. "I'm in support of whatever works, no matter who is doing it."

* * * * *

"There's some political pressure, no question," Kathy Erickson/Seitcher said when asked to comment on current relations between the cultural partners at Ka Ka Wis. "Ownership of the program has always been a source of some tension."

"When Ka Ka Wis began there were no native counsellors," she recalled. "Now almost all are native, except on the administrative side....But just to see it as cultural tension oversimplifies the situation. There are other strains as well in the program because of growth, because of change."

What is essential, she emphasized, is that "Ka Ka Wis continue to be client-centred and operate as a Circle". If a future director had an open outlook like Pat Koreski, Kathy felt, "it wouldn't matter who was in power. Because the staff would always feel that they owned the program too. Their input always would be respected."

* * * * *

While the debate about the present and future shape of Ka Ka Wis continued, the partnership enterprise went on serving client families session by session. This regular schedule was temporarily interrupted at the March-April session in 1993 when a "haunting" was reported at Ka Ka Wis. Client occupants in two family units said they had seen ghostly apparitions in "blackrobes" on the former school grounds.

Native elder Stanley Sam of Ahousat was asked to come to Ka Ka Wis and "cleanse" the haunted premises. He in turn invited Frank Salmon, Oblate pastor to several coastal communities, to join him in this operation. Frank agreed. So the native elder and the Catholic priest collaborated as each in his own way prayed and blessed the premises where the hauntings had occurred.

Frank Salmon recalled that once before the two men, again at Stanley Sam's invitation, had collaborated after an incident at Ahousat. According to Frank, Elder Sam "does not see any conflict between the Indian understanding of the spirit world and the Christian understanding".

Nor does the Oblate priest see any conflict. "In fact, the haunting by evil spirits in a lot of the Gospel stories is described in ways that are similar to the native perspective.... Anyway, we blessed all the units so I hope the problem ended there."

Does this unusual form of intercultural co-operation, described in such a matter-of-fact way, augur well for the Ka Ka Wis Centre? Is it a hopeful sign that this bridge-building partnership will continue to stand, whatever stormy weather cultural and political tensions may bring tomorrow?

* * * * *

Counsellor George Atleo has the last word in this survey report of how nearly 20 respondents assessed the future of the bridge called Ka Ka Wis. "Many of the things we have developed here are very useful for our spiritual needs, our cultural needs, our native traditions and rituals," the associate program co-ordinator said.

"Ka Ka Wis has enlightened me personally," he continued. Daily staff and counselling experiences have "made me understand my own spirituality, my sexuality. Ka Ka Wis has helped me accept myself and has helped me to develop relationships with others."

Overall, how does he regard aboriginal-white relations? "There's no way of ever severing ourselves" from the majority culture, he replied. "It's possible to have a cultural identity alongside others. We have to live alongside one another in order to have a life." — August, 1993

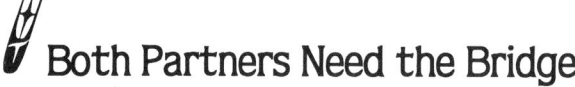 Both Partners Need the Bridge

By P.K.

One of the persisting hopes of social workers, social justice advocates and many others is that ways will be found to break the cycles of violence and abuse and injustice that many persons and different groups of people have been experiencing for generations — among them the aboriginal peoples of the world. In order for this ever to happen I believe both the oppressed and the oppressor have to become involved.

Healing – Experienced and Shared **123**

There is no doubt that the majority society has inflicted all sorts of oppression on First Nations people. If my belief that both the oppressed and the oppressors have to be involved is true, then, ironically, the partnership between natives and non-natives at Ka Ka Wis offers an opportunity for healing transformation to members of the majority culture. Those of us who come from this dominating culture can ask for forgiveness by our actions, by making amends to the oppressed culture — our native brothers and sisters.

I also believe the existing cycle of violence and injustice presents a further real danger. Native peoples could enter from the oppressor side if the healing is not done in partnership, is not done together. This is one reason I believe Ka Ka Wis is a model not only of family healing but also of community and society healing. Therefore I hope the present bridge between our cultures will hold, for the good of both, and in some small way for the benefit of all peoples — white, red, black or yellow.

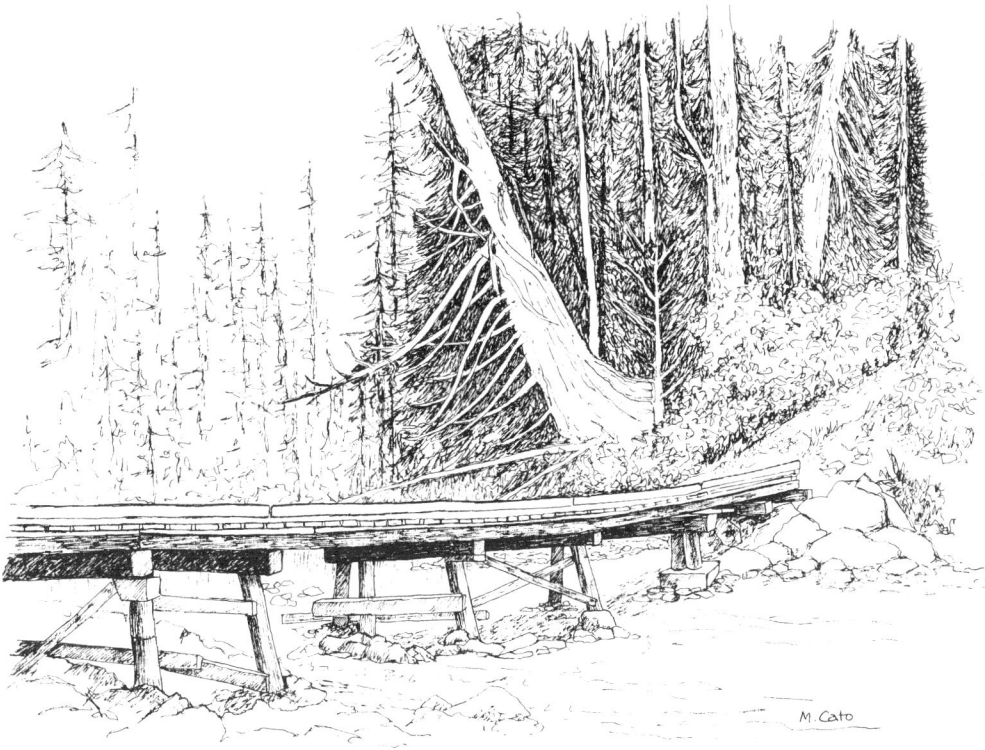

A Fragile Strength

By P.K.

For many the Ka Ka Wis Family Development Centre is a place, or more accurately, a "Circle" of strength and support. People who come here for help as well as to visit receive special gifts that make their lives better and encourage them when they feel weak and vulnerable. So one would imagine that Ka Ka Wis must be a very stable, balanced and powerful agency. Ka Ka Wis must be a well of unending water for thirsty people. The truth of the matter is, it isn't, and yet it is. Ka Ka Wis is a paradox.

From the beginning, Ka Ka Wis' strength has been its fragility, its poverty. The need for policies and a structured program grew out of the tragic death of one of our first clients. Also, in the early years our poverty was evident in the meagre facilities, budget and minimal staffing. Today we have modest but comfortable and adequate facilities, a very workable budget and a full complement of staff. So surely now we have reached a very stable and assured position. Not so. We are still very fragile and suffer from doubts and frustrations.

What is our poverty today? Ourselves. Most of us in the Ka Ka Wis Circle, if not all of us, are "wounded healers". Some of us are victims of abuse, or abusers, or both. And as much as we work on these issues and hurts, they still flare up and bring pain from time to time. It is somewhat easy to give advice and know many of the answers; it is another to put this into practice. As staff, we struggle with our own deep shame and guilt and hurts and conflicts. We struggle with working at Ka Ka Wis and walking with others in pain when our own pain sometimes feels too heavy to bear. And in our brokenness we struggle with each other. It is not easy working at Ka Ka Wis and the desire and/or real need to leave does come.

So will there always be people willing and able to work at Ka Ka Wis in our brokenness? This is our biggest unknown, our present fragility. But out of this uncertainty comes a need to trust and pray and take one day at a time, just like the people who are coming here for help have to do. "Professionals" sometimes come and find this fragility, this brokenness too hard to accept and go away criticizing or bewildered.

Perhaps one day we will all go away for whatever reason. But one thing is certain; it has been good for many of us, staff, clients and visitors. Thank you, Great Spirit, "Naas", for working through our weakness. But you should know, sometimes it is no fun at all.

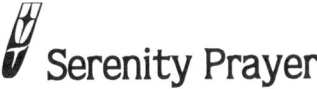
Serenity Prayer

*"God grant me the serenity to accept
the things I cannot change,
The courage to change the things I can,
And the wisdom to know the difference."*

At Ka Ka Wis you are visually reminded of this familiar prayer. You see it on inside walls and outside on a large rockface. Sometimes you will hear the verse quoted. And after almost all daily program sessions you will be invited to join in saying the Serenity Prayer.

The prayer made famous by the Alcoholics Anonymous movement certainly "fits in" with the Ka Ka Wis experience. And it applies equally to the other major challenges we face in the journey called life.

126 *Healing Journeys*

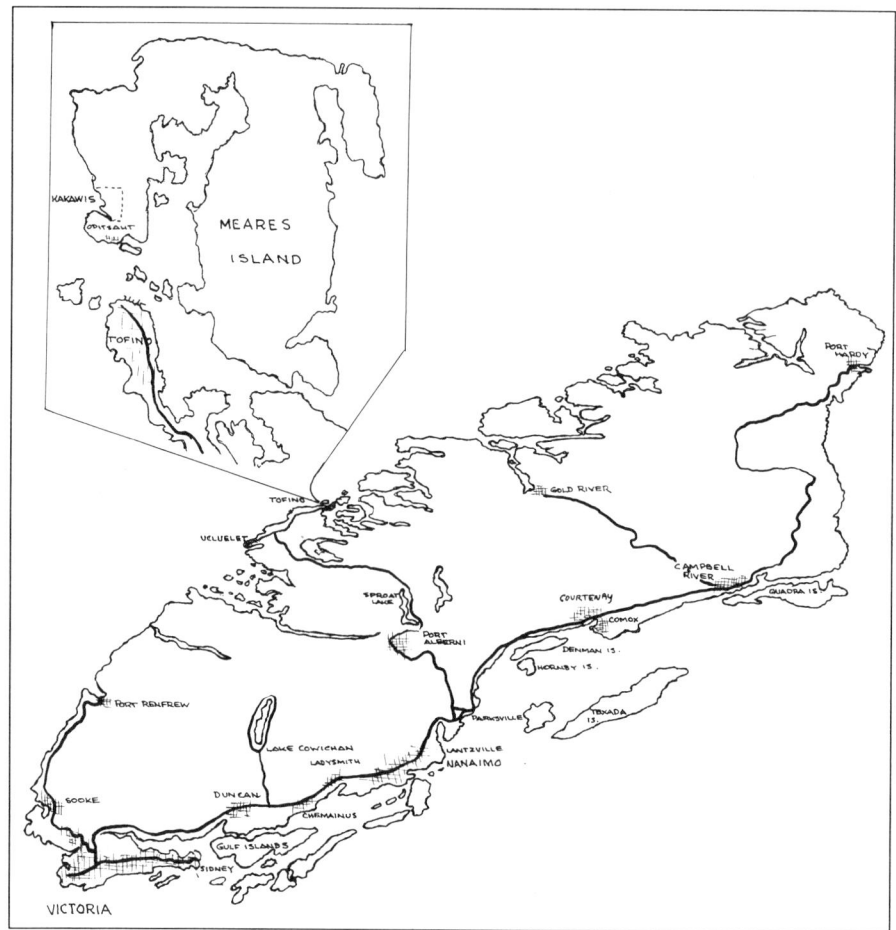

By Bob Cato

The Bigger Picture: Where Ka Ka Wis Fits in

I – Aboriginal Families – The First Pioneers

Thousands of years ago — no one knows exactly how many — the ancestors of today's First Nations peoples settled along the Pacific coastlines of Vancouver Island, Washington and Oregon.

"The land has been ours for thousands of years," said Elder Stanley Sam of Ahousat in a 1993 interview. He was referring to the Nuu-chah-nulth tribes who, as that aboriginal name says, live "all along the mountains" of the Pacific coast and elsewhere in the western half of Vancouver Island. "We know this because we still have old songs that go back for 20 generations. When the Europeans came they didn't even ask us. They just took over our land."

This native oral memory, kept alive by stories passed down generation by generation, is confirmed by the evidence archeologists unearth in their many "digs" throughout North, Central and South America. The more tribal artifacts they find, the more inclined these scientists are to say that indigenous peoples have been living in the Americas for many more centuries than first supposed.

Time magazine, for example, reported in its May 3, 1993 issue that there now is compelling evidence to believe that the first aboriginals crossed from northeastern Asia into today's Alaska and travelled on southward "not 11,500 years ago but 20,000 or 30,000 or even 50,000 years ago".

The Aboriginal Peoples of British Columbia: A Profile, published in 1992 by the Ministry of Aboriginal Affairs, opts for a conservative estimate: "Canada's first peoples have flourished for at least 12,000 years. About 5,000 years ago, more stable settlements began to emerge and increasingly complex cultures developed in all areas of British Columbia." Seven tribes representing about 70,000 members lived on the west coast of the mainland and the western islands some 200 years ago, according to this account. The Profile report continues:

"On the coast, the abundance of natural resources plus a temperate climate combined to allow the development of another rich and complex culture. In

The Bigger Picture: Where KaKaWis Fits In 129

many areas, family lines descended through the female, although this was not always the case. Property interests, held and managed by the head of each lineage, included house sites, berry, hunting and fishing grounds, as well as names, crests, songs and secret knowledge.

"These were transmitted through a ceremony known as the potlatch. Important people were invited to witness the transmissal. During the ceremony, family histories were told and the continuity of lineage established. The host of the potlatch would use the occasion to display his wealth and present gifts to the guests. The greater the value of gifts, the greater the prestige gained by the host. Although the claim to positions in society could be inherited, it was through the potlatch that rank was assumed and maintained."

These customs and the distinctive artistic expression of West Coast peoples were supported by the resource-rich coastal environment. Nuu-chah-nulth tribes became known as "the cedar people". Their long houses, boats, totems, and many domestic utensils and attractive crafts were fashioned from the western red cedars that grew along sheltered coves or a short distance up river. Some of these giant sentinels, centuries old, towered up to 200 feet above the native settlements. (Cf. ***The Canadian Encyclopedia***, 1988 by Hurtig Publishers, Vol. II, p.1318; Vol. IV, pp. 2243-44)

* * * * *

The earliest known contact between west coastal natives and whites occurred when Spanish ships twice anchored in Nootka Sound in the 1770's. A century later another keeper of oral memories was retelling old stories about the Spanish visitors. An elder named Ksagsota shared what he had learned with Father Augustin Brabant, the first priest to open a Catholic mission on the coast in the 1870's.

When still a child Ksagsota heard of the Spaniards from his grand uncle, who described a "Sunday house" where the visitors knelt, crossed themselves and sang hymns. Ksagsota had learned one of the hymns and could recall a line or two when he passed on his memories to the priest from Victoria. (Cf. Charles Moser, OSB, ***Reminiscences of the West Coast of Vancouver Island***, 1926. Or consult a more recent edited account by Charles Lillard, ***Mission to Nootka***, 1874-1900, Gray Publisher, Sidney, B.C., 1977.)

* * * * *

The provincial *Profile* report estimates that 100,000 Indians lived in what is now B.C. when the first Europeans reached Vancouver Island's western shores. Fur trading between the two cultures "increased the wealth" of some native communities, but tragically also "brought diseases, firearms and alcohol" into all native settlements. Reportedly, tribal warfare also took its toll of lives up until the middle decades of the 19th Century.

* * * * *

The local tribe always has been the main social unit of community self government. In recent years local bands have been joining area-wide tribal councils. According to the the 1992 *Profile* report, the Nuu-chah-nulth Tribal Council (NTC), with headquarters in Port Alberni, that year represented 5,745 natives belonging to 14 First Nations. The 14 tribes: Ahousat, Ditidaht, Ehattesaht, Hesquiaht, Kyuquot, Mowachaht, Nuchatlaht, Ohiaht, Opetchesaht, Tla O Qui Aht, Toquaht, Tsesaht, Uchucklesaht and Ucluelet. The tribal council publishes a newspaper *Ha-shilth-Sa* (Nuu-chah-nulth for "interesting news"), which, true to its name, is very informative.

* * * * *

Today the main occupations of the 14 tribes are troll fishing, fish processing, logging, tourism and a growing network of local social services and political structures. Culturally, especially among young people, there is a widening interest in native language and spiritual traditions.

Evidence of this cultural reawakening is seen in every issue of native publications. In its March 31, 1993 issue, for example, *Ha-Shilth-Sa* carried a report on a language conference in Port Alberni. Two elders described what they had learned from an earlier generation of elders at a meeting place known as "Paawac". From the news account:

"Elder Moses Smith said that Paawac literally means 'nest' in the Nuu-chah-nulth language. It was built of planks and it had the appearance of a nest. It was very prevalent in Ahousaht and Kyuquot. The elders sat there to 'chew the fat', said Moses.

" 'Any young person could go there if he had a question,' Moses said.... 'Paawac was very respected by the young people. I never saw kids go in there and play

The Bigger Picture: Where KaKaWis Fits In **131**

there.' He hoped this old traditional way of passing on knowledge could be revived in some way....

"Stanley Sam said 'That's where I learned what I know today. I learned it in two tribes, the Tla O Qui Aht and Ahousat. They said it was not a place to play. Be very quiet and learn what you can.

" 'Today the potlatch is the greatest teaching of our Nuu-chah-nulth,' " said Stanley. 'Only it's not really called potlatch. It's called hahts-hooltha. That's what Paawacs taught about. It taught us to use our own names.

" 'The Paawacs, that was the most interesting part of my life,' " Stanley says, 'learning from those elders. They were sharing with each other what they knew. That's the way our people educated themselves.' "

Lewis George, former native resource person at Ka Ka Wis, shared another traditional teaching with readers of the *Ka Ka Wis Star*:

"Many generations ago, our Grandparents would always make sure that our children were prepared to meet sleep with happiness. Each night they would tell our children stories about life. When the meals were prepared, the Uncles of the families would always speak to the children so they would digest their teachings as they ate.

"This was how our children received discipline. Our Grandparents told stories and legends about the animals' survival amongst themselves. There was always a moral to complete each of the stories.... It was strongly felt by our Grandparents that the children should receive these teachings so they could carry on a good and honest life.

"This teaching is still carried on today and is still used by our Elders to teach our children. This, my friends, is the translation of 'Himwitsa' "

* * * * *

The mainline media — newspapers, magazines, radio and cable networks — and also the religious media are giving increasing coverage to news and comment about the revival of cultural and spiritual practices among First Nations peoples. One of many recent examples: The December, 1993 issue of *Ecumenism,* published by the Canadian Centre for *Ecumenism* in

Montreal, featured seven articles on its year-end theme, "Past Visions & Future Dreams of Native Spirituality".

Late in 1993 the Canadian Conference of Catholic Bishops was one of several national church organizations that presented briefs to the Royal Commission on Aboriginal Peoples. One excerpt from the brief, as reported in the *B.C. Catholic* (Nov. 22-28, 1993):

"There is much in the historical relationship between the Catholic Church and aboriginal peoples to celebrate and build on. However, we are currently very aware of what was lost and this is of great concern to us.

"What was lost, or nearly so, was the free expression and celebration of the spirituality of the first peoples of this land. This weakening of the spirit of the native peoples was the most profound loss at the heart of the more obvious losses of native culture and land.

"This has been a loss for the native people, but it has also been a lost opportunity of enrichment for this country and our Church. As our North American culture becomes ever more consumed by materialism, we are profoundly in need of learning the values from the wise spirituality of the original peoples."

* * * * *

While cultural renewal is evident, economic poverty, social violence and political powerlessness remain grim realities for many thousands of Canada's first citizens. Reporting in the *Globe and Mail*, Dec. 30, 1992, Rod Mickleburgh wrote:

"Natives are more than three times as likely to die a violent death before the age of 65 as non-natives and about twice as likely to die of any cause before 65, according to a study published in the latest issue of the Canadian Journal of Public Health. Broken down into categories, the depressing litany shows the chance of homicide deaths among natives is five times the non-native rate, the fire death rate is more than six times that of non-natives, the drowning rate is four times as high and the rate for both suicide and death from a motor vehicle accident is about 2.5 times as high...."

* * * * *

The Bigger Picture: Where KaKaWis Fits In **133**

Three damning statistics sum up the intolerable situation many west coast families find themselves in — thousands of years after their ancestors first arrived in search of a better way of life. Today, Nuu-chah-nulth leaders report, First Nations tribes occupy only **one per cent of the land area**, even though they make up **half of the population** in the Clayoquot Sound area. And among these descendants of the region's original settlers, **unemployment is as high as 70%.**

No wonder then that alcohol and drug addiction, family abuse, and high rates of accidental death and suicide are other cruel realities coastal tribes struggle to overcome. And no wonder they lobby for self-government, just land settlements and other inherent rights long denied them. The only wonder is that First Nations peoples have been so patient for so long!....But for how much longer?

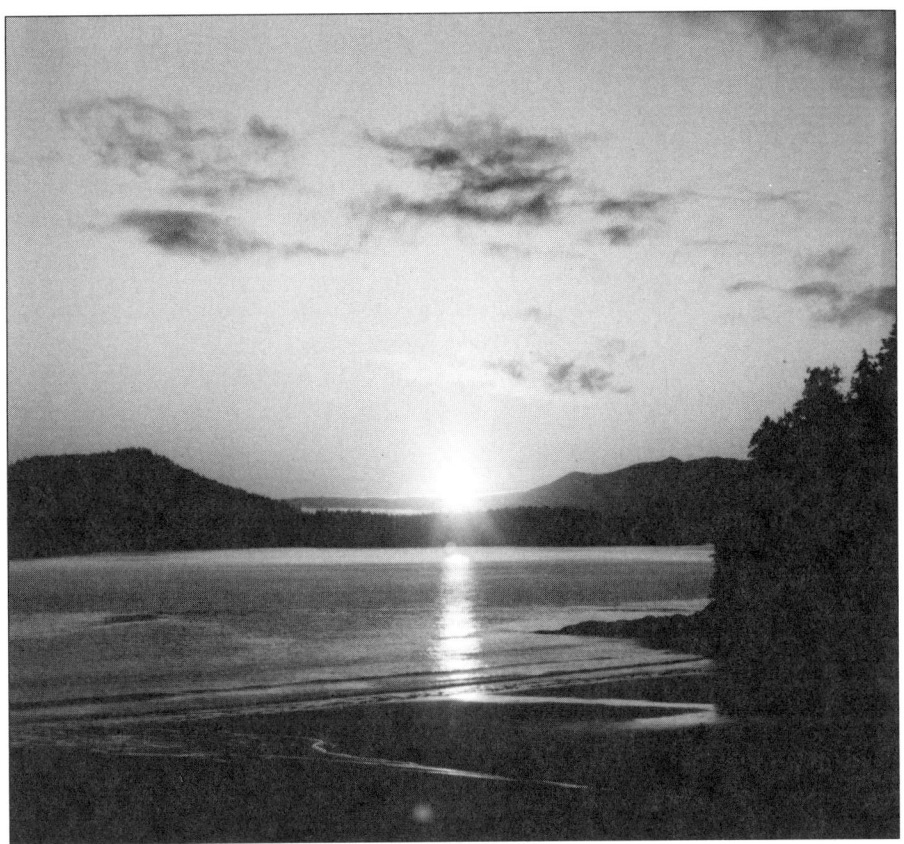

II – Christian Missions and Christie School 1874-1971

This period of the coastal saga began three decades before the first Christian mission opened on the western shores of Vancouver Island. In 1846 Rome set up the Catholic Diocese of Victoria. Its vast mission territory took in Vancouver Island, all adjacent islands, mainland British Columbia, the Yukon and Alaska!

On being named to the new diocese, Bishop Modeste Demers was heard to say, "Today...I have no clergy, no home, no cathedral. The lumber for the cathedral is still in the trees of the forest." The fledgling bishop left at once for Europe to recruit priests. He did not reach Victoria until 1852, nearly six years after his appointment.

In 1858 the Sisters of St. Ann opened St. Ann's Academy for girls in Victoria. Priests and brothers of the Oblates of Mary Immaculate (OMIs) later were given charge of St. Louis College for boys. More than a century later Oblates and St. Ann sisters were among key pioneers in the first years of the Ka Ka Wis Family Development Centre.

Bishop Charles Seghers and Father Augustin J. Brabant, aboard the schooner "Surprise", visited Pacific coastal native settlements for the first time in April and May of 1874. In his diary the priest listed the number of children he baptized at each port of call. An example: "April 26 - Baptized 177 children. I commenced at 9 o'clock in the morning and it was 5 o'clock in the afternoon when I got through..."

Less than a year later Seghers assigned Brabant to open the first west coast mission at Hesquiat. The bishop's instructions were expressed in 14 points. Three of them: "First let the missionary devote himself chiefly and directly to the salvation and spiritual progress of the Indians.... Besides these, however, let him not neglect... the temporal well-being of the Indians and their civil organization.... He shall endeavor to provide some social entertainments by which the Indians may be weaned away from indulging in their old-time native dances."

Brabant and four men manning trading posts were the only known whites living along Vancouver Island's Pacific coastline. The newly arrived priest found his isolated existence difficult. No words could describe "how lonesome one would feel were it not for the thought of the sacredness of the object for which he is here," he wrote in his diary.

But after two decades on the Pacific Rim, Brabant had overcome most of his first negative impressions. "Our Indians all over the coast are well disposed," he penned in 1895. "The people of Hesquiat, with the exception of some old men and women, being Catholic, and most of them very exemplary."

* * * * *

"After mature reflection" in 1895 the pioneer missionary wanted to "build in a central part of the coast an industrial school for boys and girls." He asked Bishop Joseph Lemmens to approve "the idea of a boarding school for our children." Both the bishop and the federal Indian agent in Victoria responded positively. But later Brabant was told to abandon the idea. Brabant was very disappointed. He still believed a boarding school for native children "is the only means to save the fruits of my labours of more than 20 years."

A few years later Bishop Alexander Christie reversed his predecessor's decision. Christie wrote to Brabant: "I want to consult with you about building a boarding school for the Indian children of the west coast. I have just returned from Ottawa and have obtained a per capita grant from the government for 50 children. If we do not accept the grant it will be given to one of the sects...."

Augustin Brabant hurried to select a site for the new school. He chose well, picking a location that later was described as "neutral ground" outside the territories traditionally occupied by different tribes. Some aboriginal elders believed it had been a "sacred place" in earlier times. The priest had practical considerations in mind when he chose a site on the shores of Meares Island that would be "easily accessible to all the Indians on the coast." Moreover, here Mother Nature had provided an awesome abundance of resources. Brabant's description of the location:

"At the foot of a mountain (now known as Lone Cone) in Deception Channel I found and secured a large piece of table land open to pre-emption and away from all Indian settlements. It is 50 feet above the surface of a fine bay which at low water has a sandy beach of more than 20 acres — a magnificent playground for the children. It is also in proximity to another bay, a real clam field, so that with a bay swarming with salmon and other fish and a large field of clams, the expense of supporting the children will be considerably reduced and their health will be benefitted...."

* * * * *

The first school buildings — a 60 by 40 ft. two-storey structure and a small outside laundry — were built by October 1899.

The first staff invited to operate Christie Residential School were American Benedictines. Four men and three women left Mount Angel, Oregon, on May 7, 1900. They reached the wharf in Clayoquot Sound nine days later. On May 29 the school opened with Father Maurus Schneider, OSB, as principal. The other Benedictines were Father Charles Moser, Brothers Leonard and Gabriel, and Sisters Mary Placid, teacher; M. Francis, cook; and M. Clotilda, seamstress and dressmaker.

Only 10 pupils were present that opening day. By July, 28 were enrolled and another 16 came later that first school year. Language differences were not the only or even main reason for the limited response. "It was hard to get the children," admitted Moser, later the school principal. "The parents did not like to part with them. It needed a lot of coaxing and persuading."

* * * * *

By 1900 schools for aboriginal children had existed in Canada for three centuries. In 16th Century New France, as Québec was then known, mission schools were operated by the Recollet, Jesuit and Ursuline orders. In the late 1700's and early 1800's Anglican and Protestant schools also began teaching native pupils elsewhere in Canada. By the time Christie School opened, federal government policy had been promoting boarding schools for young natives for 70 years. By 1900 there were 64 residential schools operating across the country. They were part of the determined federal policy to assimilate Indians into Canada's then nearly all-white society. By 1922 Ottawa was vigorously enforcing the Indian School Act, which decreed that all school-age aboriginals must attend designated schools.

* * * * *

Two anniversaries were observed on Meares Island in 1925. Charles Moser described them that December: "In August of this year we celebrated at the Christie Indian Residential School amid a great concourse of Indians from all our missions, the 50th Anniversary of the establishment of the first mission at Hesquiat in 1875; and the 25th Anniversary of the opening of Christie Residential School." There were 80 children then enrolled as 1925 ended — including "the 167th boy and the 154th girl that entered since the school opened."

The double anniversary observances in 1925 provided "new impetus" to act on Brabant's first published accounts of his years on the coast. In 1900 a religious journal in New York published his serial account of his mission experiences. Soon bound copies of the series were in demand. When Moser succeeded Brabant as pastor of the Hesquiat mission in 1910, the Benedictine priest resolved that one day he would republish Brabant's story along with a report of his own later experiences. After the double anniversary celebrations Moser did so in *Reminiscences*, published in 1926 by the Acme Press of Victoria. Today the book is an invaluable source of information about missionary events and attitudes as one century was ending and another beginning.

* * * * *

In 1938 Frs. Hildebrand Melchoir and Leo Walsh, the last Benedictines to have charge of Christie School, were recalled to their home monastery in Oregon. Canadian Oblate priests and brothers replaced their American predecessors. George Forbes, OMI, the incoming principal, together with Fr. S. Sorensen and Br. John MacDonald, OMI, arrived "on the First Friday of August, 1938".

Christie School celebrated its 50th year in 1950. Observances to mark this golden jubilee included publication of a special edition of *The Tillicum*, the school journal. It is a revealing document — in what it tells and in what it neglects to report, in who contributed comments to its pages and who did not, and in the opinions expressed.

The booklet featured nearly a dozen individual articles and accompanying photographs. All writers were male, all were white, and all but two were Catholic priests. Evidently, not one word was contributed by a native person, male or female.

Although positive comments about native students were expressed, only one of the anniversary reflections was directly addressed to aboriginal readers. Fr. Victor Rassier, OSB, who had been principal in 1929-35, wrote: "My dear Indians: It was my happiness to spend five years working in your midst....As I look back over my life, I can truthfully say that those were the happiest years in my life. You called me Friend, and showed by your conduct that you spoke that blessed word from deep down in your hearts."

Some viewpoints expressed by the unnamed author of a lengthy article:

"In needlework and embroidery the girls have always been among the first in Provincial Exhibitions. The penmanship of the boys and girls has been widely acclaimed.... The first graduates of the Palmer Method of writing were Joseph and Savey Tumtum and Peter Brown of Nootka Sound.

"The school has also proved to be a melting pot for the different tribes along the coast. Every tribe is well represented and a spirit of friendship exists between the different coastal tribes today. Years ago the different tribes were continually at war with each other. The school and the missionaries have done more than their share in destroying the tribal enmities."

"The first children who came to the school (in earlier decades) ...did not know what the future held for them," wrote Fr. James P. Mulvihill, principal in 1941-47. *"They were leaving the carefree life of their villages to be cooped up within four walls where everything would be planned for them according to 'white ways' and where their liberty would be sacrificed for a few added comforts."*

By the 1930's, however, Mulvihill continued, "the majority of children came from homes where the parents had also been school graduates....Instead of mistrust and obstruction, the parents, who have the greatest influence with their children, advised them on entering school to take advantage of their stay to learn all they could and benefit by the example of those dedicated to God...who were working for their salvation and happiness."

* * * * *

After nearly six decades at Christie, Benedictine sisters were suddenly recalled by their Oregon superiors in 1959. That September they handed over their teaching and domestic duties to members of another American society of women religious — the Sisters of the Immaculate Heart of Mary.

(Forty Benedictine women served at Christie from 1900 to 1959. In 1974 sisters from the same Oregon community returned to Vancouver Island, settling in Nanaimo, where today they maintain the House of Bread Monastery and operate the Bethlehem Retreat Centre. As for the Immaculate Heart sisters, members of their order have been teaching native and other children, first on Meares Island and now in Tofino, ever since they came to the area 35 years ago.)

The new arrivals in 1959 were popularly known as "the Hollywood nuns" because they hailed from Los Angeles. Sr. Peter Damian, IHM, headed the new feminine staff. Accompanying her were Srs. Ruth Anne and Juan Diego — the religious name chosen by Marie Cooper of Saanich, the order's "first Indian vocation". The three Benedictine sisters they were replacing — Colette, Alexander and Leona — stayed until June, 1960 in order "to show the ropes" to the newcomers.

Michael Kearney, OMI, Christie principal, welcomed the California sisters. Besides their duties at the residential school, the IHM sisters agreed to help out at the day school at Opitsat, the neighbouring reserve community on Meares Island. Opitsat was one of four missions then served by Tom Lobsinger, OMI.

Magnificat, published by the IHM order, in October 1961 featured an article on their new apostolate on Vancouver Island. The unnamed author described the Christie program and offered some impressions of the student body. An excerpt:

"Because of their poverty and lack of opportunities, it was considered a feat for an Indian child to complete the eighth grade. Within recent years, however, many have gone on to high school. Some have taken vocational training, and many have obtained good jobs. But most of the boys return to the reserves to take up the work of their fathers — fishing. As for the girls, since most of them marry soon after leaving school, it is important that they be trained in the domestic arts....

"From the time they recite their morning prayers until the day ends with night prayers, the Indian children are steeped in the Christianity the missionaries brought....The boys and girls are under the care of the priests, brothers and sisters 24 hours a day, nine months of the year."

* * * * *

By the early 1960's "Old Christie" was one of 65 residential Indian schools operating across Canada under religious auspices. Of these, 42 were Roman Catholic, 15 Anglican, six United Church (formerly Methodist) and two were Presbyterian. Twelve of the schools were in B.C. Native students then living in residence numbered over 10,000. The federal Indian Affairs Department provided public funds based on enrolments. In the mid '60's, for instance, Christie School received about $650 annually for each resident student. But times were changing; by 1965 the majority of aboriginal children in Canada were attending day schools.

June, 1971 was a memorable month for Christie staff and students. The school closed its doors after seven decades. That year the Indian Affairs Department opened a new residence in Tofino to house native students. Beginning that fall they would attend public schools in Tofino and Ucluelet.

At Old Christie two days of closing ceremonies in June attracted native families, the well-known elder and film star, Chief Dan George; three bishops and other clergy, plus various educational, civic, provincial and federal representatives. One of the participants was Larry Mackey, OMI, Christie principal for most of the 1960's.

In a 1993 interview he said the closing events brought "hundreds of native families to Meares Island. There were dozens of native boats anchored in the bay in front of the school. It was quite a sight." Harry O'Connor, OMI, the last principal, was master of ceremony. Also on the program were members of the Native Advisory Board, which Mackey had organized when he was principal. Some original members of this advisory board, he recalled, included Louie Frank, Barney Williams, Sr; Nelson Keitlah, Sr.; Moses Smith and Alex and Louise McCarthy.

* * * * *

The Bigger Picture: Where KaKaWis Fits In   141

Three to four generations of First Nations children and youth resided at Christie School during its seven decades. How many students were there in the 71 years? Complete records were unavailable when preparing this overview. But an "educated guess" seems possible. Based on annual attendance figures for one or two years in each of the seven decades, total registrations at Christie may have been around 7,000. But according to an Oblate source, total individual students likely numbered around 1,500. The two very different totals are not really incompatible, since most students would have been registered several times — once during each of the school years their names were on the Christie roll call.

* * * * *

In 1990 Fr. Tom Lascelles, Oblate archivist in Vancouver, offered a carefully balanced response to critics who claimed residential schools in past decades had been "little more than brutal prisons" for native students. In a 100-page study, *Roman Catholic Indian Residential Schools in British Columbia,* Lascelles offered his assessment of the record. He did not directly address the much discussed issue of abusive treatment, sexual or otherwise. Part of his appraisal:

"Early missionaries, like most members of their society, had little appreciation of native cultures, and even less of native religions. In those days, too...native peoples were not asked what kind of education they wanted their children to receive. Through the schools, moreover, the churches to a degree became instruments of the goverment's policy of assimilating the Indian people into the dominant white society, a policy the government vigorously pursued for several decades. Native children were gathered by the missionaries, or by Indian agents and constables, and taken to residential schools. There they were educated according to foreign standards. There, too, children were obliged to speak English, and sometimes were punished for speaking their native language....

"Today's missionaries acknowledge the offences that have been committed, endeavor to benefit from the lessons the past teaches, and seek to be instruments of peace and healing with those who have been wounded by their or others' insensitivity....

"Native peoples' brokenness...however did not begin and end in the residential schools. It stems rather from a multiplicity of sources, alcohol being among the most pervasive since the days of the fur trade era, and one that has steadily undermined the people's spiritual and cultural values....

"And if alcohol is not noxious enough, the tides of injustice, discrimination and unemployment, to name but a few, induced further brokenness".

* * * * *

In 1991 the Roman Catholic Diocese of Victoria completed a five-year Synod process, called by Bishop Remi De Roo to chart policy guidelines for the future. Among the 400 "decisions for action" approved by Vancouver Island delegates at weekend assemblies were 14 policy recommendations on aboriginal issues. One dealt with residential schools. It read: "Offer, as a Church, an apology for the damage and pain caused by the institution through the boarding school system and try to have a public reconciliation with members of native villages as part of an ongoing healing process."

Three Postscripts to the Christie School Story

1 – Students' and Teachers' Memories

Twenty years have passed since the Ka Ka Wis Family Development Centre replaced and gradually "transformed" what had been Christie School. Memories of residential school days at "Old Christie" or elsewhere still are fresh in the minds of many former pupils and teachers, including some native staff, board members and clients of the present Centre.

These school recollections surfaced quite often during interviews in 1992-94. Here are some representative comments heard during these conversations.

- Tommy Curley, part time staff member at Ka Ka Wis, was at Christie in the 1940's. "I really had bad feelings for a long time," he said. "When I first went there I couldn't understand why I couldn't speak my own language. Why was I separated from my brothers and sisters? I couldn't talk to them and this made me feel bad.

"A lot of resentment also came because you didn't have your parents to talk to and give you support. Every day when you learned something new, you wanted your parents to know about it but you didn't have that....To this day I have mixed feelings."

- "Apart from having to leave my mother and dad and the grandparents, it was pretty good at Christie," Florence Frank, now of the Toddlers' Learning Centre, recalled in describing her experiences from the late '50's to the mid '60's. "The teachers were really strict but I learned lots." Florence most regrets having to give up her native language, which she now tries to recover.

- "The language rule wasn't our rule. That came from above....It bothered me every time I had to say, 'Speak English'." Sister Justine Zollner, OSB, 76, shared this painful memory of her teaching years at Christie in 1940-48 and 1956-59.

  She was in her early twenties when she first faced more than 30 native pupils in grades one and two. "I wasn't well prepared.... I had never taught primary grades before. I didn't know the native language and most of the children didn't know English. I depended on some second graders as interpreters."

  Difficult as she found it, Sr. Justine saw that it was much more trying for the grade one pupils. "It was totally foreign to them. Some were so bewildered, so homesick. So I tried to be a little mother to them."

- Rose Tom, who helps tend small children at the Ka Ka Wis Toddlers' Centre, was at Christie in the 1950's. "I hated it," she said emphatically. "I used to go home (to nearby Opitsat) on Sundays. My parents had a hard time getting me back there."

- "Sure, there was the real pain of separation for both parents and the kids," acknowledged Tom Cavanaugh, OMI, a staff member from 1964 until Christie closed in 1971. "But it was the wish of most parents that their children come to Christie," as they themselves had done.

  As disciplinarian of the male students, he followed the norms common to schools at the time. Sometimes punishment for serious misconduct was a strapping, and other times some student privilege was denied. "I don't think we were too severe."

What about allegations of sexual abuse? "I didn't see anything as far as staff was concerned," Tom replied.

- "Residential school prepared me for life outside" in the mostly white society, Marie Donahue, Centre counsellor said. "Racial prejudice was foreign" to her growing up in a native community. "But our teachers at Port Alberni high school prepared me for that. So I was ready to handle prejudice when I encountered it later on."

- Sister Roberta Dyer, OSB, replaced Justine Zollner in 1948 and stayed until she was recalled to Oregon in 1954. "I volunteered. I'm an adventurous spirit... and I have some Indian blood myself," said the 75-year-old Benedictine. Like Justine before her, Roberta taught grades one and two together — as many as 40 pupils some years. The two-way language barrier meant "I didn't get any learning into them until March and April" of the school term. The children's drawing and carving skills particularly impressed her.

  Roberta and Justine visited Ka Ka Wis in 1992. Later that year they welcomed about 15 graduates of Christie, representing three generations, who made a return visit to the Benedictine monastery for a special "Ka Ka Wis Day".

- "I didn't like Christie much — the way we were treated," said Loretta Williams, briefly a day-care assistant at the Learning Centre. "I found out how mean some teachers could be.... If we didn't eat, they saved the leftovers for our next meal. One woman lay teacher used to hit us on the head with her stick or grab our ears."

- Chief Francis Frank of the Tla O Qui Aht First Nations tribe, lives at Opitsat, next door to Ka Ka Wis. He has become widely known as an eloquent champion of native interests and rights in the Clayoquot Sound environmental disputes. Chief Frank was a pupil at Christie from the middle '60's until its closing. What was his experience there?

  "I had no problem with it, actually," he answered. "It was a good experience for me." Did his learning there contribute to his adult leadership skills? " Undoubtedly," he replied.

The Bigger Picture: Where KaKaWis Fits In **145**

- Howard Tom, Tla O Qui Aht band manager, has positive and negative memories of his six years at Christie in the 1940's.

  "Compared to most, I never had that much difficulty," he said, and then added: "But there was too much religion and we lost our native language, even though I didn't know a word of English when I started.... Overall, my experiences there were quite good and I learned discipline."

- In 1959 Immaculate Heart of Mary Sisters from California replaced Benedictine Sisters at Christie. Ever since then, Sr. Anita Tavera has been one of several IHM members who have taught native children — first at "Old Christie" and later in Tofino. She described a typical day at the residential school, from early rising to night prayers, including recreation time. "The kids were very creative in their play because there were very few toys. They liked sports, weiner roasts, putting on plays and the like... We treated the students as if they were our own."

- "Compulsory attendance was a requirement of the Indian Affairs' education branch. It was something beyond our authority," Larry Mackey, OMI, stated in recalling his years as Christie principal in the 1960's. "English was the language of instruction....But I never laid down any rule as to what language students used outside the classroom."

  In retrospect, Larry Mackey felt the Oblates "took the heat" for school policies and rules made by Ottawa and the B.C. department of education. "The trick the government used was the per capita grant. You needed more students to run the school in order to get enough money to feed and clothe them. It was a 'Catch 22' situation....Native parents had every right to complain about the whole process!"

- Probably Barney Williams, Sr. spoke for many other former students of residential schools when he described how he felt about that past experience. In February 1991 he was one of 13 aboriginal elders invited to address mostly white Synod delegates representing the Catholic Diocese of Victoria.

  "I was more or less raised by Oblate priests and Benedictine sisters at Christie and I count some clergy among my personal friends," he said. "But that doesn't make me agree with the way white society and missionaries once approached our people.

"When I was a little boy, the missionary would come to take us to school, and my brother and I would hide because my father told us, 'They want to take you away'.... He didn't understand what the missionaries were trying to do and they didn't understand him either.

"But today I feel we now understand....Let's heal this for our children so they can stand with their heads high."

(Cf. **Forward in the Spirit, Story of the People's Synod**, 1991, pp. 184-88)

* * * * *

A similar emphasis on the cultural effects of residential schooling was noted by an observer who represented the Catholic bishops of Canada when the Royal Commission on Aboriginal Peoples met in Canim Lake, B.C. in March 1993. Jennifer Leddy noted that the complaints voiced at the meeting about sexual abuse in residential schools received extensive media coverage. But, Ms. Leddy pointed out to a CCN reporter, "the prevailing concern among the aboriginal people who were there was about the impact of these schools on their culture, their language, their whole sense of alienation."

* * * * *

2 – Paint the Whole Picture!

By P.K.

When I first came to Vancouver Island in the late '60's I was on holidays. Through some unusual turns in the road I ended up on the shores of Old Christie School. I remember my arrival very well. It was a beautiful summer day. Reg's sound system was in full swing and Jim Reeves was singing out of the trees. Lots of kids were on the beach playing in and out of the water. I spent a wonderful three days and thought I had visited one of the happiest places in the world.

I still remember the party that was sort of thrown to honour my friend and me. There was lots of singing and laughing and games. I especially remember a big, quite strong-looking man who quickly figured out a difficult puzzle game we were playing, but said nothing. His name was Pat Little. He and his wife Vera were on staff. Actually, I remember all of the staff who were there, and how welcoming all of them were to my friend and me....Reg O'Brien most of all.

I visited Christie each summer in the next two years. Then, on my third visit, I answered a job opening and was accepted on staff. I started work at Old Christie on Meares Island in August of 1970. I believed I was joining a very happy team doing marvellous work. Happy to be working so hard to provide something special and good for a group of students. There was a sense of pride and dedication among the staff. The long hours and little or no pay were offset by the good that was happening.

How things have changed, and hindsight has smeared my beautiful memories. I was part of that system for five years. I met and married my wife at New Christie in Tofino. Today, when speaking to strangers I am very reluctant to acknowledge that I was there. Especially when I'm talking with "educated" social workers who have read and therefore know all about the "despicable" experiences, but who were never really there to see for themselves at firsthand.

As I write this, deeply buried feelings are coming to the surface. I would like to say this, then: When the whole system is condemned lock, stock and barrel, remember Reg O'Brien and the others like him who dedicated their lives to helping children grow up in this world and have a better future. Look in his face and then, if you can, pull the trigger.

I can easily accept that there were many wrongs in and about Christie. At Ka Ka Wis we deal with this almost daily. You don't know how much I want to apologize for those wrongs and my part in them. My working at Ka ka Wis is one small way of doing that.

But God!, I wish some of the leaders (like some of the people, in quiet, do) would stand up and thank those who really did think and strive to do their best. I wish some of the leaders would stop painting a completely one-sided picture. I wish politics the hell out off the scene! And I wish the media would begin reporting the whole story.

I don't believe full healing will ever be possible until both sides are heard. But who am I to say this? I am one of the guilty.

3 – Towards a Balanced Viewpoint

By G.A.

I cannot help but note that as I write this a workshop is being held in Port Alberni on residential school experiences. I attended a residential school in the 1960's. It was both a good and bad experience. Much is being said today about the bad experiences.

But for some students, residential school also was a safe place to get away from family issues happening at home. And a lot of what we learned there has helped many of us ever since. I hope what is said here will enable some readers to reach a more balanced view of the residential school experience.

My grandmother, father, mother, uncles, aunts, brothers, sisters and cousins attended residential schools. Though little was said about their experiences, a lot didn't have to be said. They lived it daily by sharing the skills they gained by attending residential school.

A very strong statement that holds true for many is made when they witness the rich and vibrating sounds of a saxophone played by an uncle, a piano played by a grandmother, a guitar played by an aunt, an accordion played by a father, and a harmonica played by a mother. Or when witnessing with awe the handwriting skill of my grandmother, father, mother, aunts and uncles. And when seeing the creative and artistic talents of those who developed skills they now share with others. It may be in sports, sewing, operating and maintaining a boat, or home cooking, or the discipline of getting up early for daily chores. Or consider any one of the many other abilities and habits a person may have acquired by attending a residential school. These are the kind of strengths and skills that we all can build on to further develop the life styles of our communities.

One of my happiest school memories is of a warm-hearted man on staff who shared his beef, lettuce and tomato sandwich with us during our evening snacks.

III - Ka Ka Wis: Healing Circle for Families 1974-94

The new story of the Ka Ka Wis Development Centre began to unfold almost as soon as the Christie School story ended. The Family Development Centre idea was first conceived, took shape during a long pregnancy, and came to birth in early 1974. Looking back over the 20 years since then, director Pat Koreski identifies the Centre's three stages: the growing-up years before 1984, the middle period when the family focus sharpened in 1984-89, and the maturing years when the "healing circle" widened in the early 1990's.

1 - The "Growing-up" Years Before 1984

1971 - What Now for "Old Christie"?

Should the Oblates sell the vacated school property? Or might the 70-year-old buildings be used in creative new ways?

'71 Highlights — That July a visiting Jesuit challenged members of religious orders to listen to west coast native people and support their dreams for Ka Ka Wis.

- In October Jim MacDonell, Oblate pastor at nearby Tofino, moved to Ka Ka Wis to manage the school property until its future was decided.

- Native groups and others offered many suggestions: Start an adult-education centre to give school-upgrading, teach technical skills, boat-building, arts and crafts. Arrange a summer camp for children and youth. Provide a retirement home for Indian seniors. Begin a program to help aboriginal clients deal with family breakdown and its causes, especially alcoholism.

Who Were There — Besides Jim MacDonell, fellow Oblate Gerry Guillet, pastor to several coastal reserves, often was at Ka Ka Wis between boat trips. His United Church counterpart, Rev. Lloyd Hooper, visited when he could. Reg O'Brien, by then maintenance manager at the new Christie Residence in Tofino, also spent spare time at Ka Ka Wis.

Comments Then & Later — At an early planning meeting an aboriginal parent declared: "It's no use just sending the one who is drunk for treatment. The whole family has to go."

- Jim MacDonell: "The idea was that if the natives came up with a reasonable program, we would use the buildings for that.... Many natives were interested once they knew they had a say in what was going to happen."
- Louie Frank, educational leader in Ahousat: "Right from the closing of the residential school the Oblates were ready to move on whatever we might want to use the buildings for....I know there's a lot of negative talk but I've always found the Oblates willing and open."

1972 – The Search Continues

More voices were heard in the widening debate about what to do at Old Christie, where a small core community and support group maintained the premises until decisions were made.

'72 Events - The Kyuquot tribe, headed by Chief Kelly John and Jackie Leo, band manager, pressed for a Ka Ka Wis program that would help families cope with home problems. Mary Lou John, wife of the chief, pushed for alcohol rehabilitation.

- The Kyuquot community was thought to have less alcoholism than other coastal reserves. But a new study indicated over 90% of Kyuquot households were affected by drinking in some way. Dr. Iain Kenning, psychiatrist and director of Victoria's Eric Martin Institute, visited Kyuquot with Gerry Guillet and Lloyd Hooper to discuss this report with native leaders.
- A small team was organized to visit reserves and sound out more aboriginal views on Ka Ka Wis. Larry Mackey chaired the travelling group.

Who Were There — Martin Saxey, once the breadmaker, boatman and all-round handyman at Old Christie, often visited. Irene Leo came on weekends to share her cooking skills. Curious holidayers and people seeking community — among them adult Christians and youthful hippies — came to Meares Island. Most "culled themselves out" and moved on.

Comments Then & Later — Many possible uses of the buildings at Ka Ka Wis were listed in a letter written by Chief Kelly John on behalf of the

Kyuquot band. Ideas included: Hold AA meetings. Teach courses in plumbing, electrical work and other trades. Offer a small-business course. Organize "evening entertainment with NO BOOZE". Teach volleyball, baseball and other games. Bingo. First aid. "Help retarded children or others behind in learning." These activities "could give employment for a lot of our Indian people at the old school. They'd probably feel right at home there...Try to keep open all year. Have three or four groups come for three months at a time."

- Dr. Kenning said he was impressed during working visits by the determined way many natives on Vancouver Island dealt with alcoholism. "They had identified the problem, were working at it and achieving some changes. I guess the Ka Ka Wis development is an early example of that."
- A native mother's reasons to stop heavy drinking: "I don't want to pass on the habit and disease to my five kids. I want to be an example to them and show them I don't need a crutch. My only high will be feeling good about myself."

1973 – Decision: Start a Family Centre

Full agreement was reached on "a plan originating with the west coast native people".

'73 Happenings — In February the Ka Ka Wis search team held inquiry meetings at Ahousat, Kyuquot and Opitsat. Over 90 people took part in the events, sponsored by the Nootka Fisheries & Cultural Society.

- **A Ka Ka Wis memo described the consensus: "All the communities without exception want Ka Ka Wis to be reopened....One community put the reasons in writing. They want Ka Ka Wis to be a counselling centre for families... 'a home away from home'."**
- Soon a program plan was ready. Known as "The Kyuquot Proposal", it described a "Kakawis Family & Community Development Project". Several prepared the project plan, among them Chief Kelly and Mary Lou John, Band Manager Jackie Leo, Billy Cox, Jacqueline Woodford, and Oblate priests MacDonell, Guillet and Mackey.
- A charismatic retreat at Ka Ka Wis drew 70 participants. Some who came and other newcomers joined "the core community" for awhile. The pioneer staff's first draft of a counselling program began to take shape.

- So far modest funding to support the small community had come from the Oblates who maintained the former school property; the Diocese of Victoria (including a $11,500 grant from the Catholic Church Extension Society), and from the Sisters of St. Ann, Victoria, who assigned two members to Ka Ka Wis in 1973.

Who Were There — The basic community consisted of MacDonell and Guillet, Lloyd Hooper and his wife Frances, Sisters Lorraine LaMarre and Kathryn Erickson, SSA, Pat Koreski and Joe Fligstein, former seminarians, and two native families who came to give support by their presence and skills: Louie and Eva Frank and children from Ahousat, and Alban and Rose Michael from Nuchatlitz.

Comments Then & Later — From the *Minutes* of February meetings in reserve communities: **Ahousat**: "The overall response was very strongly positive, with emphasis on the conviction that... Old Christie be used according to the wishes of the people of the coast. The people also expressed the important factor of neutrality of the land at Old Christie — not belonging to any one Band, but rather to all the people of the coast..." **Kyuquot**: "Expressed desire for Christie (again as 'neutral ground') to remain open and used in some educational capacity for all the people of the Coast...." **Opitsat**: "Voiced agreement with the reports of the two previous meetings."

- "Louie and Eva Frank, with their children, came to share their life with us that first year," Lorraine LaMarre recalled. "Louie continued his seasonal fishing and transported his children to Tofino school every day in his troller.... That winter had many hardships — many rain and wind storms.... The Franks contributed much to community that first year." (1981 memoire)

- Eva Frank: " It was good living there when we did. The program does help people but a few fall back, and there's still a lot of drinking. My husband and I never had a drink. We just never had it when we were growing up."

- "We lived a really shared life," Lorraine remembered. "We prayed, worked, talked and played together. We didn't have much money so our life style was very simple." Kathy Erickson/Seitcher agreed. The pioneer staff "had to rough it", whether unloading heavy supplies from their boat, or

The Bigger Picture: Where KaKaWis Fits In **153**

sharing blankets with the Frank family to keep the cold winds out of their living quarters. "When the winds blew, we used to say that the termites held hands to keep the old buildings from falling. But our spirits were high."

- Bishop Remi De Roo, Victoria, was encouraged by what he saw happening: "It's a venture in faith.... If there is a response to a real pastoral need, and if the Holy Spirit wants it that way, it will survive.... You have to admire the fortitude and spirit of the priests, sisters and Indian families who are willing to launch this project and see what happens." (*B.C. Catholic,* Dec. 5, 1973)

1974 – Good News and Sad News

The first native clients came to Ka Ka Wis for counselling. That was the good news. (This new beginning would be celebrated 20 years later in 1994.) The sad news was that a woman client died there in 1974.

'74 Highlights — In May nine clients — three couples and three single men — arrived from Gold River, Kyuquot, Hesquiaht and Port Alberni seeking help. Later, two of the couples and one of the single men joined the support staff.

- A tragic incident that claimed a life happened in early November. A woman client and her two preschool children were living at the Centre. One night her husband arrived by boat, bringing liquor. Drunkenness, quarrelling and her accidental death followed.
- In response the Ka Ka Wis staff prepared a code of conduct for resident clients and family members.
- Dr. Kenning gave a four-day workshop on Transactional Analysis for the fledgling staff. "He gave us the necessary confidence and we organized formal counselling sessions," Lorraine LaMarre said.
- The new Centre asked the B.C. Ministry of Human Resources for $175,429 to set up an ambitious counselling program. No answer came. Later on a scaled-down request for $46,429 was refused.

Who Were There — Brother Tom Cavanaugh, OMI; Sister Mary McGarrigle, SSA, a registered nurse and former hospital administrator; and Marjorie Kuntz, CSJ, also a nurse, joined the core team. "Extended community" members included Ray and Sarah Williams, Archie and Ruth Little, John Lucas and Russell Joseph.

Comments Then & Later — Jim MacDonell: "There was a period when things looked very doubtful in '73-74. I remember Bishop De Roo came up for a visit. We didn't have any clients at the time, funds were scarce, and sometimes we wondered whether to pack it in. The Bishop encouraged us to hang in a little longer. He thought the Centre was a good idea and needed time to jell....Also, Monsignor Mike O'Connell was a significant supporter in those days. He visited us and gave us moral and financial support. He had a very caring attitude and presence."

- KA KA WIS REBORN AS SYMBOL OF LOVE. This headline in the July 13, 1974 *Victoria Times* topped a story by Humphrey Davy. "A unique family counselling centre, believed to be the first of its kind in North America, has been established on a secluded island situated five miles north of Tofino", the story began. "It is unique in that parents with their children take up temporary residence at Ka Ka Wis....The counselling centre differs from similar services operating in cities where people are counselled or treated as individuals apart from their families."

- Lorraine LaMarre: "Kathy and I did much home visiting that first year, getting to know the people and trying to start the catechetical program. We went to Ahousat twice a month for several days at a time, where we lived in an Indian home loaned to us by Pete and Lil Charlie, who were living in Victoria managing a group home for boys. We learned how to live without electricity, how to cope with sooty oil stoves and roaring gas lamps and packs of dogs, and other less challenging things." (1981 Memoire)

- Mary McGarrigle, SSA: "We had very little to live on, we were isolated, but I loved it all! After hospital administration, it was a relaxing time for me. Everyone there was kind and considerate... Tom Cavanaugh kept us well supplied with fish he caught.... There was real community, which you didn't always find in a religious community."

- Frances Hooper: "Well, it was different there. There was a tremendous feeling of co-operation. It was a very happy time."

The Bigger Picture: Where KaKaWis Fits In **155**

- "The Ka Ka Wis gang" extended an open invitation in the December *Newsletter*: "The Old Christie school buildings still shake before the onslaught of gusting southeasterlies and westerly gales. But do come and visit us. We have plenty of room and are cosily housed. Come on a Friday evening to enjoy our weekly community meal and get-together in a big kitchen which now has the homey sound of a wood fire crackling in the huge black 'used-to-be' oil stove. Or come any evening to enjoy some music from the piano and guitar...or to enjoy card games, Yahtze, or a game of pool. Or join us in the gym for a volleyball game, or bowling in the homemade alley!....Come and celebrate Eucharist with us daily in the historic old chapel, which is the centre of our community."

1975 - A North American First

This continent's (and perhaps the world's) first residential counselling program for native families began at Ka Ka Wis.

'75 Events — Sixteen clients, married couples and a few single adults, from Kyuquot, Port Alberni, Chemainus and Duncan lived at the Centre while taking part in the first session. Their school-age children attended classes in Tofino, where most stayed week nights at the New Christie residence. On weekends they rejoined parents and younger family members on Meares Island. Clients and staff looked forward to having school classes at Ka Ka Wis.

- Jim MacDonell and Lorraine LaMarre travelled regularly to Victoria for training seminars in Transactional Analysis.

- In October the B.C. Alcohol & Drug Commission approved a first grant of $14,888 to help Ka Ka Wis operate for the next half year. Monthly statements and regular progress reports were required. This first public funding and prospects of more financial support lessened the Centre's dependence on previous sources.

- In 1974-75 six native families and three single men "lived at the Centre for varying lengths of time, received some help by counselling, and contributed much to its growth", the Ka Ka Wis Newsletter reported.

Who WereThere — The small community of staff and supporters now included the Girvans — Archie, his wife Katherine, and three sons. Plus the Petersons from Port Alberni — Jack, an electrician, and Yvonne.

Comments Then & Later — Lorraine LaMarre recalled that in 1975 Transactional Analysis was "our main tool. We also recognized the need for AA and prayed for a recovering alcoholic to come and live here and be part of the program. In August our search was rewarded when Archie and Katherine Girvan came to live with their three sons...Archie is a non-status Indian...(who) has 10 years of sobriety and forms an active part of our program through his voluntary work with AA-based counselling. This couple was well suited because they did not mind the isolation and were not overly concerned with financial security, which no one could offer at this stage...." (1981 memoire)

- The Ka Ka Wis *Newsletter* listed developments the staff hoped "to see happening" soon. Two such hopes: See more native people getting involved in the operation of the Centre, "directly and indirectly, in the roles of management, counselling, advisory, etc." And see that after leaving Ka Ka Wis, more client families would "help their own people in their villages and in cities by sharing what they had learned with others, and by sharing their strength with others."

1976 – Step by Step

By late 1976, 26 aboriginal families, including 86 children, had enrolled for counselling since the program had begun.

'76 Happenings — Dave Hawkes, elementary school principal in Tofino, headed efforts to get federal funds so a teacher could be hired to instruct clients' children at Ka Ka Wis.

- The Centre received increased funds for 1976-77: $66,480 from the provincial A & D Commission and a $29,000 Local Initiatives grant from Ottawa.

- A "volunteer Board of Directors" was chosen to administer funds: Roy Haiyupis, Clayoquot band member, chairman; Gertrude Frank, community health worker from Ahousat; Darlene Haubrick, public health nurse; Tofino's Mayor Don McGinnis; Dave Hawkes, school principal; Hugo Peterson, former Tofino mayor; Linda McConnell, Gerry and Lorraine.

Who Were There — December roll call: Gerry Guillet had switched his main residence from Tahsis to Ka Ka Wis, where he joined fellow Oblates MacDonell, Cavanaugh, and Frank Salmon, the new Catholic pastor of Tofino,

Ucluelet and Ahousat. St. Ann members LaMarre and Patricia Donovan. The Hoopers — Lloyd and Frances. The Girvan family of five. Also Ray and Sarah Williams and family some of the time.

Comments Then & Later – "We are trying to have the whole family change its pattern of living," Lloyd Hooper told the area newspaper, *Westcoaster*, that January. If alcoholic members were to achieve sobriety, other family members also had to change their ways, he emphasized.

- Reactions of two clients after Ka Ka Wis counselling: "You know, I feel a lot better. But we're still in the same boat — still alcoholics," said the first. "Well, I know what makes me tick anyway," the second said. (*Alberni Valley Times*, May, 1976)
- A later survey report by two social scientists praised the work of Centre staff: "The steady devotion of the pioneers... laid a foundation which would remain.... They developed the program, hosted dozens of visitors, did the books, and cleaned the six client units between sessions. The capable hands of Reg O'Brien were always on call as well." (Drs. Evelyn W. Pinkerton and Dr. Eugene N. Anderson, *The Ka Ka Wis Experience*, 1986, pp. 11-12)

1977 – "Getting it all Together"

A serious shortcoming in the residential program was overcome when school funding arrived.

'77 Highlights — Thanks to the efforts of Principal Dave Hawkes and others, minimal federal funds arrived so that Ka Ka Wis could hire Virginia Vandean to begin teaching school-age children that September. Sr. Pat Donovan cared for preschoolers and taught Parent Effectiveness Training (PET) to mothers and fathers.

- The annual grant from the ADC was $77,640 for 1977-78. Another $11,580 was received for outreach work among former and prospective clients.
- By September, 50 adults, accompanied by over 50 children, had participated in the program since October, 1976.
- Gerry Guillet, on six-month leave, visited addiction treatment centres as far east as the Quebec border. His United Church colleague, Lloyd Hooper, followed doctor's orders and retired to Saltair with his wife Frances.

Who Were There — Besides the Centre team and native families living at Ka Ka Wis, others came for counselling from Dawson Creek, Shalalth, Lillooet, Enderby, Agassiz, Mission, Chilliwack, Burnaby, Vancouver, Duncan, Kuper Island, Nanaimo, Port Hardy, Harrison Lake, Kyuquot, Gold River, Bella Bella and Opitsat.

Comments Then & Later — The fall *Newsletter* welcomed the first Ka Ka Wis school teacher, Virginia Vandean, to "a bright new classroom".

- Patricia Donovan later recalled, "I think in that first year Ginny didn't take her full salary because she wanted some of it to be used to buy school equipment." Lorraine agreed. "She bought a lot of equipment that first year." And the salary itself was "very minimal". (Taped recollections recorded in 1985)

- "I did buy some supplies but I don't think I spent a tremendous amount," said Virginia, now Mrs. LeJeune of Agassiz, B.C. She described the experience as "a mixed bag but I did enjoy it." Class size ranged from five youngsters to nearly 20 in very small quarters.

- "Each day is a new day in which we can turn to our Higher Power and ask for help," the Centre *Newsletter* reminded client readers struggling to stay sober. A quotation followed: "When I pick myself up after falling for the third time this week, I remember not so much that I have fallen but that I have picked myself up. For today, that is sufficient."

- From a September report: "All (clients) have maintained sobriety while here and have left with a determination not to drink. Maintenance of this sobriety, however, has often proved difficult. We believe the following negative elements are to blame, and not an ineffective program nor an individual's lack of responsibility, as one might suppose: undue pressure by drinking relatives and friends bearing on extremely sensitive and dependent natures (formed by culture and environment); few opportunities for selective choice of activities and friends, due to isolation of villages; lack of understanding of alcoholism and of supportive systems, such as AA...."

1978 – Ka Ka Wis becomes "Official"

Without giving up its informal ways, the Centre gained legal status during the year.

'78 Happenings — The Family Development Centre was registered as a non-profit body under the B.C. Societies Act. Serving as the first official Board of Directors were Stanley E. Douglas, RCMP; Don McGinnis, contractor; Geri Seinen, nurse: Olivia A. Mae, business person; and Gerry Guillet, priest.

- Oblates MacDonell and Guillet shared duties as joint Centre directors during the late 1970's. Each took leaves of absence to rest or study.
- Three two-person teams worked with client families during six-week sessions. Lorraine and Gerry conducted morning TA sessions. Larry Mackey and Patricia Donovan handled video taping and play-back reactions from the clients. (Fr. Mackey's stay ended when doctors advised him to give up the physically demanding life at Ka Ka Wis.) Ray Williams and Wilfrid Andrew led the evening AA meetings. Meanwhile, at the Learning Centre Janis McDougall succeeded Ginny Vandean in September.

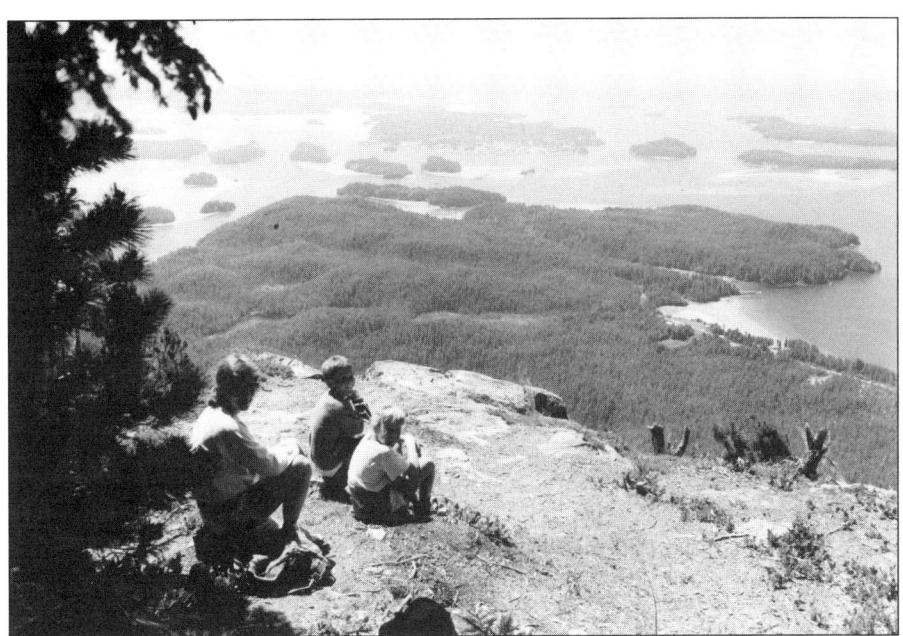

- The Centre's boat, the "Remi J.", blew up and burned — fortunately without injury to anyone. The June *Newsletter* said a "bouncing new, blue-eyed boat" had already replaced the stricken vessel.

Who Were There — Mostly the same crew as before plus the Andrew family from Friendly Cove — Wilfred, and some months later Margaret Andrew and their children. Wilfred had achieved sobriety before arrival and Margaret would while at Ka Ka Wis. The Andrews were to live there for seven years — lending a hand in counselling and in many other ways.

Comments Then & Later — "It was a good experience for all the family," Wilfred Andrew said in summing up seven years of residence. But both he and Margaret agreed that the Centre had "a different feel" when staff no longer lived on Meares Island, but instead commuted daily from Tofino. In any case, after living there several years, Margaret said it was time "to get out and see what it was like outside. I felt really secure there and had all the protection. I was too comfortable, too safe."

- "I would consider going back if a teaching position became open," Janis McDougall remarked when describing her teaching days at Ka Ka Wis. Class size ranged from three to 18, and pupils' ages from kindergarten years to mid-teens. With older students she concentrated on remedial English and mathematics.

1979 – Changes, Growth and Growing Pains

The Centre was in transition as the Seventies ended.

'79 Events — In June Jim MacDonell said farewell after eight eventful, often stressful years as director or joint director of the Centre. He moved on to another Oblate assignment at Chemainus.

- An independent team assessed the Centre program for the provincial A & D Commission. The examiners found that program ideals were high and the quality of counselling good. More outreach work was required in native communities. Understaffing was named as another problem, along with the need to upgrade some staffing skills and bookkeeping records. Objective criteria were needed in order to measure the program's long-term effectiveness.

The Bigger Picture: Where KaKaWis Fits In **161**

- Edwin Frank and Gertrude Frank, native representatives, joined the Board of Directors.

    Comments Then & Later — Poetic tribute to the departing Oblate was paid by Centre colleagues. Some lines:

    "Farewell to McTavish — our Nova Scotian friend.
    Let your future bright and restful be....

    He came here to stay eight years ago.
    Lonely and cluttered was this place....

    Not a day went by but that something broke down:
    T'was the boats, the ramp, the water, the power,
    The truck, the tractor, the 'phone, the float!
    He was often discouraged to the point of giving up hope.

    He cleared the place of junk, burning many a pile.
    There's much he demolished; much he has built;
    New apartments he named, a Board of Directors,
    And a Family Development Centre worthy of fame."

- Ray Williams, pioneer client and later a counsellor and all-round handyman, continued to spend some time at Ka Ka Wis.

1980 – Gerry at the Helm

From mid-1979 to June 1984 Fr. Guillet continued to be a key figure on the Ka Ka Wis team. As two visiting consultants later observed, he "stamped an indelible mark on the program".

'80 Highlights — Some former client families returned for four seven-day "renewal" sessions during July. Overall, there were 63 family admissions in a 12-month period.

- "Misfortune struck again... when the 'Ave Maria' sank at the Tofino dock," Patricia Donovan reported in the March *Newsletter*. A freight-passenger boat, the "Ave Maria", first had served Christie School and then the Centre. But all was not lost. As the Newsletter went on to report: "We managed to have it lifted but we are still waiting for the engine to be repaired. Joe Kranabetter from Tofino has been giving up each Wednesday afternoon to transport the families back and forth to do weekly shopping."

- The first new living unit was constructed in 1980-81.

Staff News — Carol Sadler taught clients' children for one year. She would return in 1987 and continue as lead teacher at the Learning Centre in the 1990's. Valerie Bob became Outreach worker and Newsletter editor when Pat Donovan returned to Victoria after serving four years.

1981 - Birth of the Blue Bead Ceremony

The original Blue Bead Ceremony took place in August at the first annual Sunrise Celebration. Ever since then the bead service has marked the climax of each counselling period.

'81 Happenings - Two 6.30 A.M. sunrise ceremonies on Sunday and Monday mornings of the long August weekend climaxed a three-day "celebration of sobriety" at Ka Ka Wis. It was sponsored by the Centre staff and supported by AA groups from coastal reserves, the regional tribal council, and visitors from the Round Lake Centre. The three-day event included an opening ceremony, welcoming dance, speeches, prayer circles, a Mass of thanksgiving, visits to the sweat lodge, singing and drumming, a Potlatch with barbecued salmon, healing sessions, and the first Blue Bead service. The weekend focus was positive throughout. Everyone knew alcoholism was killing good people, Gerry Guillet said. "We wanted to show all the good things that also are happening."

Staff News — After eight years of round-the-clock service. Lorraine LaMarre was transferred. Sister Patricia Shreenan, SSA, replaced her as senior counsellor for the next four years.

Comments Then & Later — Lorraine wrote a brief history of the St. Ann Sisters' service at Ka Ka Wis since 1973 and shared some parting reflections: "What are our hopes for the future? One is to continue to be a core Christian community along with the Oblates and the families that live here full or part time."

1982 - The Ninth Program Year

"Gerry ran a mature, if young program. The staff was free to develop, improvise, create. Time was fluid, energy unlimited. Volunteers provided much

The Bigger Picture: Where KaKaWis Fits In

effort. Gerry himself set the tone...." So wrote Drs. Pinkerton and Anderson, social scientists, in their later report. (Cf. *The Ka Ka Wis Experience*, p. 15)

'82 Highlights — In January the B.C. minister of health received a brief on "Upgrading Safety and Health Standards at Ka Ka Wis". The appeal for funds to renovate the 80-year-old premises was submitted by Pat Koreski, then chairman of the Board of Directors. Supporting letters from native leaders and Tofino supporters were included. The appeal was heard: a small supplementary payment was followed later by a larger annual ADC grant of $185,914.

- The upgrading brief cited some 1975-80 totals for the Centre's counselling program: 81 two-parent and 17 single-parent families, plus 17 single adults, had taken part in the residential sessions. Overall, nearly 500 were involved — 205 adults and 277 children and youth.
- All Board directors were reappointed for another year except the retiring chairman, Pat Koreski. In October Gerry Guillet began sharing his duties as director and also his salary with Pat, who became administrator.

Staff News — Brother Reg returned to live on site, where he had first resided from 1950 to 1971. Sister Margaret Cantwell, SSA, arrived to begin teaching at the Learning Centre in the new year.

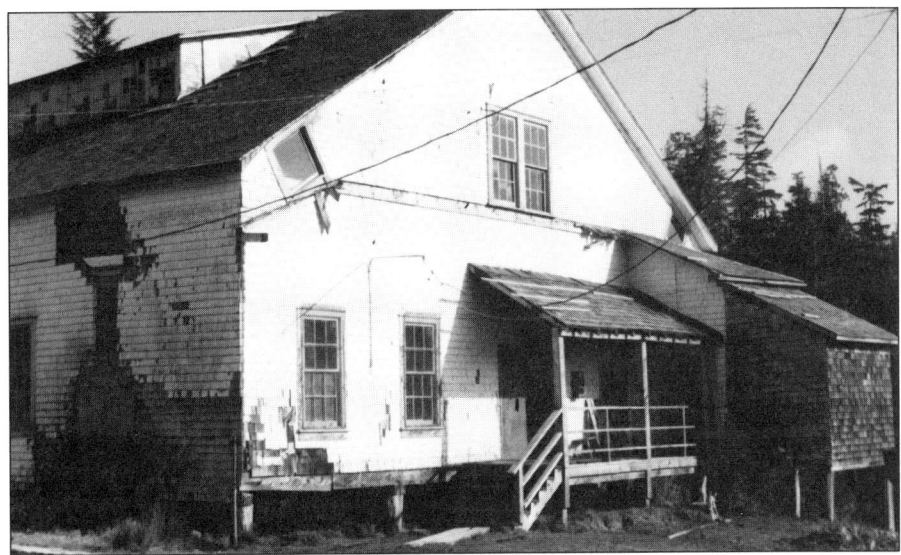

Comments Then & Later - Fred Miller, OMI priest-journalist, writing in *Home Missions*: "The people who make it (Ka Ka Wis) work are the 482 people who had the courage and the will to get the necessary help to rebuild their lives that were out of control due to alcohol. Energized by their example, there is a steadily growing list of families waiting their turn." In future, he predicted, Ka Ka Wis "will be seen as one authentic witness of the Gospel in action."

1983 - The Fire and a New Beginning

The Centre's growing-up years came to a fiery end one summer night. Symbolically, the ground was cleared for new chapters in the Ka Ka Wis story.

'83 Happenings — July 15 was the night Old Christie burned. Four families and four staff workers living in the main building lost possessions but escaped unharmed. Numbing shock, concerns and hopes were experienced there and far beyond.

- John James led a morale-boosting workshop as staff and volunters began to clean up and rebuild. A round-the-clock team effort meant that only one six-week session had to be cancelled because of the fire. Sessions resumed in large trailers.

Staff News - Program director Gerry Guillet was also visiting pastor to Long Beach, Opitsat, Tofino and Ucluelet. His double work load was taking its toll.

- Margaret Cantwell, Learning Centre facilitator, also edited the new *Ka Ka Wis Star*, an expanded newsletter prepared by both clients and staff.
- Sr. Patricia Shreenan, SSA, compiled a 10-year survey of families who had completed one counselling session.

Staff News - Two couples — Mabel James, the new day-care director, and Joe Hnasiewich, maintenance worker; and Bob and Maureen Cato, active "retirees", joined the Centre team.

Comments Then & Later — A native parent was one of the early clients to tell her story and share her thoughts in the expanded newsletter: "When I was 14... I left home on my own. My Dad kept drinking. He sank lower and lower. My brothers grew up. They drank. I drank. I never stopped crying. Then

I had children of my own. I hurt them the same way my Dad hurt me. At Ka Ka Wis I learned all the hurt I carried had to be set free. Now it's over and gone. I'm myself. I'm me. I made mistakes. And my children understand."

2 – Sharpening the Family Focus 1984-89

1984 - New Directions

The Centre's pioneer years were over and its leadership changing. A dedicated family man succeeded the dynamic priest who had been associated with the Ka Ka Wis experiment from the start.

'84 Highlights — Pat Koreski took full charge. Gerry Guillet moved on to new pastoral challenges in Hope, B.C.

- Thanks to the insight and initiative of Patricia Shreenan, the counselling approach developed by Virginia Satir was adapted for client sessions. Staff and clients became familiar with the many "hats" family members wear at different times in household relationships. They learned about "roles" in behaviour that blocked good communication in the home — from the dictating "blamer" to the apologetic "peacemaker", from the ever-busy "distractor" to the aloof "computer" member.

Comments Then & Later — "I want to encourage all those thinking about going to Ka Ka Wis for treatment," Ron Hamilton, native leader, wrote in *Ha-Shilth-Sa*. "I saw families opening their eyes to each other there, and alcoholics being healed. I saw people struggling with themselves in beautiful surroundings and I saw people helping each other with every means at hand, unashamed and unafraid." (Dec. 6, 1984)

- Roy Haiyupis also endorsed the Centre program, writing in the *Ka Ka Wis Star*. The aboriginal leader spoke to client families. He commended their "courage, strength and determination" in coming to Ka Ka Wis, then added: "I know you will go from here knowing that others need help and that you will be helping others back home."

1985 - Continuing Growth

The new captain at the wheel "brought order and thoroughness to files and finance," reported the two anthropologists who spent eight weeks at the Centre.

'85 Events — Drs. E. W. Pinkerton and E.N. Anderson came from U.B.C. and California to observe the Ka Ka Wis program.

- Three earlier staff leaders, Jim MacDonell, OMI, and SSA members Lorraine La Marre and Pat Donovan recorded Centre memories on a cassette tape for the Pinkerton-Anderson team.
- A staff-development week became part of the Centre schedule. Largely financed by the Sisters of St. Ann, six staff members attended a Satir training workshop on Gabriola Island.
- The Ka Ka Wis counselling program was explained at an Alaskan conference on "Healing the Family".
- A Canada Works grant, supplemented by the Oblates and the provincial ADP, paid for renovation of Ka Ka Wis buildings and facilities.
- The *Westerly News* featured an account of a lively November event sponsored by Ka Ka Wis. The report described a fund-raising night in the Clayoquot Sound Community Theatre. Dancers, singers, musicians, mind-readers and comedians competed for prizes.

Staff News — Pat Shreenan was transferred after four years at the Centre. Sr. Carol Proietti, SSA, had already arrived to assist Margaret Cantwell at the Learning Centre. Kathy Erickson was once more connected to Ka Ka Wis.

Comments Then & Later — After a six-year assignment elsewhere, Joe Leins returned to Vancouver Island as regional director of Alcohol & Drug Programs, Ka Ka Wis' main source of funding. He revisited the Centre and was "a little surprised and disappointed" that the counselling program had not developed more during his absence. He expressed concern to the director, who got the message. In the ADP leader's words, Pat Koreski "did a lot of work developing the program and he made Ka Ka Wis an active part of the whole Tofino community."

- "Ka Ka Wis is first and foremost a place of prayer, an opportunity for prayer," Pat wrote in the Centre paper. "I believe this with all my heart.... Working at Ka Ka Wis I find it necessary daily to turn my will and my life over to the care of God as I understand him. This is prayer and this is Ka Ka Wis."

- Some clients also shared spiritual reflections. A young woman wrote: " As a child, we had family prayers once a week, Mass every Sunday. It was confusing along with the violence....But in my 20's it was positive, as I had a wonderful husband and a good support system....Now I've grown away from anything 'spiritual' and I feel a loss, as I remember a peace within myself for a short time before."
- Centre counselling, another client said, "has given me the basic understanding of my inner spiritual self.... This has given me the foundation that I need to grow in spirit, and has renewed my faith in the Higher Power. Now I realize that I need to have faith in God so that I may nourish my spiritual inner self."

1986 — Evolving and Evaluating

The B.C. government's Alcohol & Drug Programs carried out an evaluation of the Ka Ka Wis counselling service.

Other Happenings — The Pinkerton-Anderson report, based on the two anthropologists' 1985 stay and follow-up interviews with 40 former clients, was published.

Staff News — Kathy Erickson became program co-ordinator, a position she held for the next six years.

Comments Then & Later — One of the Pinkerton-Anderson findings: "Ka Ka Wis' level of success is very high compared to most treatment programs that service North American clients. It more than meets the criterion that about one-third of clients become abstinent and another one-third improve, a rule of thumb for judging a program adequate." But the authors added that a long-term evaluation of results was needed in order to assess the lasting impact of Centre counselling. (Cf. *The Ka Ka Wis Experience*, p. 73)

- "My life before coming here consisted of two basic things, despair and alcohol," a client wrote in the *Ka Ka Wis Star*. "My life was unmanageable, I was lonely , and I was sinking in the quicksand of alcoholism." But after a reluctant start and after coming to trust her counsellor, this client saw her life and future in a different light. "I saw that I had been given a reprieve by God in the form of caring people. And I had been given a chance to live again — one day at a time."

1987 – The Audit and its Aftermath

The provincial ADP "audit" of Ka Ka Wis found "the program has now 'come of age'", having grown from "fragility to stability".

'87 Highlights — The report, written by Ann Tasko and the agency's four-man research team, said the Centre's "history of flexibility" and its newfound strength made possible needed improvements. Ka Ka Wis was described as a bridge linking "the best of traditional native Indian values and beliefs with the best of today's Western society." (Cf. *The Ka Ka Wis Program, History & Current Description*, 1971-1986, May 1987, p.74-75.)

- The *Tasko Report* stressed the importance of the group Circle used in counselling sessions and also for some class activities for children. Another observation: "Ka Ka Wis is not an alcohol treatment centre designed by government for native Indian families....It was not superimposed on the native population by non-natives. Rather, it is 'a bridge between the needs of the people and the identified problem'." (p.19)

- The Tasko findings were published in May. Later Pat Koreski circulated a brief progress report: "We have finished living through 'the Audit' and can confidently state that documentation, scheduling and reorganization have added depth to the Ka Ka Wis experience...."

Staff News — Elaine Greig became the Centre's bookkeeper.

Comments Then & Later — Duart Farquharson's reporting made headlines in Southam newspapers across Canada with his news reports from Ka Ka Wis. One observation: "Though it is not religious in a denominational sense, it invokes a strong element of spirituality — whether through native 'sweat lodge' practices, the Higher Power of Alcoholics Anonymous, or the Christian God."

- What one client wrote before going home: "A special thank you to all counsellors who have helped us through all we've learned here. Especially to Mabel James. If she didn't come over to our unit in the second week, when we were having our ups and downs, we probably would have left. Mabel gave us the encouragement to hang in there, which we did. We've sure learned a lot, especially to communicate with each other and as a family....We don't feel like leaving, but what we have learned here we can share with others on our reserve."

- The June 18 issue of *Ha-Shilth-Sa*, published by the Native Tribal Council in Port Alberni, carried a report asking for "more support and involvement" at Ka Ka Wis: "Most of the 40 people attending the Contact Persons' Workshop pleaded for more involvement from Elders and band leaders in the battle against alcohol and drugs."

1988 – The Power of the Circle

The healing power of the Circle was stressed by many clients in their comments.

Some Events — What one client wrote in describing his experiences in the Adult Circle: "Thank you all for being a part of me through the last six weeks. I got close to each one of you one way or another, and I'm grateful for being in a strong circle. You gave me the strength and courage I needed to help break down that wall and let out all the hurts, pain and anger that I've been carrying around so long. Now I could cry and not feel ashamed about it. But most of all I could laugh again and feel good about myself and others. Now I will share with brothers and sisters back home. I hope I plant a seed in some of them so that they can start on that right road to sobriety...."

- Counsellor Mabel James reported: "Maybe two or three times in a six-week session I facilitate an all-women's Circle. The first one is very heavy, as they share stories they have held back for so long. We will end with positive feedback and then do some fun together."

- The now treasured 10 by 8 ft. Dance Curtain, which symbolizes the Ka Ka Wis experience, was designed and painted by male clients at the spring session. "The message it carries is very powerful....I had a big lump in my throat when we first viewed it," one couple reported in the *Ka Ka Wis Star*.

Staff News — In Ireland, Jack Ryan, the former priest-counsellor at the Centre, who himself battled alcoholism, died of cancer. After six years at Ka Ka Wis, Mabel James left for new challenges. Before going she paid tribute to the Irish Oblate: "He was a patient teacher when I first started counselling.... He left a lot of wise words behind and from them we are able to accept his passing." Joe Tom and Daryle Blackbird began their staff association at Ka Ka Wis.

- A *"Special Hesquiat Edition"* of the *Ka Ka Wis Star* circulated after a workshop for members of that native community. Some who took part said they had more appreciation of their responsibilities as parents. As one wrote, "What we learned really shows how important mother-love and father-love is to our children. Little ones form an opinion about themselves that is based on the love they receive from others." Another stated: "I feel proud to be a mother....Although the hours are usually long and sometimes hard, I truly believe there is no other occupation more fulfilling."

- New counsellor Merv Bannon said one six-week session had been "a beautiful soul-searching and eye-opening trip" for him. "No university or higher learning institution that I'm aware of us has courses that teach what is being shown, heard and felt here, Why? Maybe because we are all teachers and students to each other."

1989 – Focus on Aboriginal Culture

A special celebration at the Family Development Centre in October demonstrated that "native culture and traditions are alive and strong at Ka Ka Wis."

'89 Highlights — A large outdoor carving on the Centre grounds and a dozen 8 by 4 ft. art panels indoors were unveiled during a "Celebration of New Beginnings". The carving of stylized land and sea creatures overlooks the wide beach. The impressive work was designed and crafted by Cecil Dawson, son of Ruby Keitlah. She and husband Nelson Keitlah hosted the event.

Staff News — Kathy Sawyer began her four years as secretary-receptionist at the Centre.

Comments Then & Later — Many clients continued to express their thanks to Ka Ka Wis in the newsletter after sessions ended. Examples: "Thank you for guiding me along my new path until I could see my own way." And: "We've laughed, we've cried, we've opened our souls. We've told our pains and told our plans. We've bickered and complained, and we've shared our joys. We have been a great Circle."

- Beginning in the late '80's, the Learning Centre qualified for public funding from School District No. 70. Funds were to be used to purchase supplies and equipment and pay salaries and benefits to staff. Denny Grisdale, Port Alberni, then district principal for First Nations' school education in District 70 (which included Tofino and Ucluelet), administered these funds on behalf of the B.C. government's Provincial Resources Program. He praised the quality of teaching by Carol Sadler and associates at the Centre. "They have a wonderful program for children of young native families," Mr. Grisdale declared. Later, his successor, Ron Erickson, was equally positive in his comments.

3 – Widening the Healing Circle 1990-94

1990 – New Tensions in Changing Times

As a new decade began, public controversies — from the Mohawk-army standoff near Oka, Quebec, to a local property dispute in Tofino between native leaders and municipal officials — increased tensions for some staff and clients at Ka Ka Wis.

'90 Happenings — A collective "profile" of 860 adult clients from 1976 to 1990 showed the male-female ratio was almost one-to-one. Average age was in the early thirties. Family size averaged 3.6 children in 1976-80, and declined to 2.8 by 1986-90. Other comparative figures for the two five-year periods showed that the percentage of common-law couples and single parents had increased while the number of married couples had declined. In 1976-80, for example, married and common-law couples were almost equal — 41% and 40% respectively. By 1986-90 48% were in common-law unions and only 27% were married.

- With professional help the Centre produced two videos to show and tell the Ka Ka Wis story. Two of the titles: "Coming to Ka Ka Wis" and "The Healing Circle". The videos are available for viewing.

Staff News — George Atleo joined the team as a counsellor trainee.

Comments Then & Later — Clients' children at the Learning Centre were sometimes asked to write on assigned topics. One such assignment topic: "What

I know about alcohol". The answer by a 12-year-old boy: "Some people die from drinking beer. First they lose their jobs. They get so drunk they go through alleys and stuff and die. They get stabbed. They throw up blood. They go to jail. They lose their homes, cars and their life....Once Mom was going to jump off the bridge but the cops came and stopped her...A lady came and said she was taking me to a foster. I slammed the door in her face. Then I locked the bathroom. The cops took me to the foster. I stayed there a couple of weeks and went to see Mom....Mom's lawyer was talking to these other people. She had to promise to go to AA and stuff like that."

1991 – Time to Widen the Circle

The Board of Directors decided a thorough program review and renewal plan were needed. So the third close examination of counselling services since the mid-1980's was carried out.

'91 Events — This review began with a definite goal in mind: Find more effective ways to "expand the Ka Ka Wis Circle" so that there would be better day-to-day outreach beyond the Centre. Foster more two-way co-operation between the Ka Ka Wis staff and their opposite numbers and client families on reserves, both before and after counselling sessions.

- With this goal in mind, the ADP's Carol J. Savage was seconded to the Centre where she spent May and June. By August she had written a preliminary report. Called *Expanding the Ka Ka Wis Circle*, the "review and enhancement" report proposed a "new program model" that foresaw three stages of recovery from alcohol or other addictions: Cleansing, which aimed for stabilized sobriety; Healing, which sought ways to strengthen family life; and ongoing permanent Recovery, by developing a healthy life style.
- This program review was financed jointly by the National Native Alcohol & Drug Program and by B.C.'s ADP service.
- To give the Board of Directors a Vancouver Island-wide representation, four women from as many areas were appointed: Wilma Keitlah of Port Alberni, Grace Neilsen from Nanaimo, Mary Everson of Courtenay, and Debbie Williams of Duncan.

Staff News — Reg O'Brien "retired" and was quickly named the "ex officio mayor" of Ka Ka Wis, where he had spent most of the past 40 years.

Comments Then & Later — "The Circle is the conceptual heart of the Ka Ka Wis Family Development program," the new assessment report recalled. It quoted from the earlier *Tasko Report*: "As with many native healing programs, the circle symbolizes wholeness, protection and equality for all those in it — bringing alive the values of caring and respect for one another."

- *Expanding the Ka Ka Wis Circle* also affirmed the *Tasko Report's* 1987 insight that saw the Centre as a bridge. "The bridge provides a crossing from a place of cultural oppression, a place of perceived powerlessness...to a place of strength and freedom".

1992 - Feedback on the Renewal Plan

In April 45 copies of *Expanding the Ka Ka Wis Circle* were circulated among First Nations' leaders and professional associates on Vancouver Island. Later, 41 of those contacted were interviewed. Their feedback provided a directional compass for the staff.

'92 Highlights — One feedback proposal said "Ka Ka Wis should tell its own story and celebrate and share its successes". This affirmed a recommendation in the 1991 renewal report: "Hold a celebration of '20 years of transformation'" that had "turned Christie into a program which helps native families to heal and to value their own spiritual teachings."

- In response to the two reports, the Board of Directors and the Ka Ka Wis staff decided to hold an anniversary celebration in 1994 — 20 years after the first clients had come to Ka Ka Wis for help with addiction. Pat Koreski invited Grant Maxwell of Victoria, a veteran journalist and author, to assemble and edit a "book of celebration" in time for the 1994 event. He agreed and worked closely with Pat, the Centre staff, former clients, Board members, and others in preparing the story you are reading now.
- Community co-ordinating services began publishing two newsletters. Former clients received *Stars of Ka Ka Wis*, while referral agencies and associates got the *Ka Ka Wis Star*, using the same name as the former

in-house letter. Editor Sherry Merk introduced a new format and a breezy style of reporting.

Staff News — Kathy Erickson, program co-ordinator and one of the original Centre staff, departed to become director of the Port Alberni Drug & Alcohol Counselling Service. Her successor as program director, David Zryd, arrived with his wife Nancy and their infant son Jonah. Mabel James rejoined the Ka Ka Wis team after a two-year absence.

Comments Then & Later — Joe Tom, community-services co-ordinator, shared the first outline of a proposed plan of action to "network elders, chiefs and councils, NTC and ADP care-givers" with the Centre team: "How can we work together for the benefit of our people? Some ideas I plan to work on: 1 - Show videos of Ka Ka Wis. 2 - Explain how Ka Ka Wis works, and how much work needs to be done BEFORE treatment....3 - Provide AFTER CARE as long as it is needed. 4 - Help ensure that skills learned are used and that new skills will be learned as families grow. 5 - Ensure that each person has a say and a choice in personal, family and community life." Joe concluded his outline with a request:"If you have any ideas, please share."

- In October senior staff were asked for their views about the proposed "book of celebration". Some replies: "Our story still is not understood by some Band Councils. It would be ideal if when they read this book they'd say, 'This is about us too.' ".... "What's the purpose? Who's the audience?" .... "It all depends on how it's handled. You can't have too much patting ourselves on the back. Be real and honest in telling the story. It's the clients who heal themselves. We just walk with them and offer some guidance. Believing in them is the key.".... "Try to send a message that we native people are trying to make a better life ourselves. Ka Ka Wis is part of the message. We promote healthy family living here and show it can be done."

1993 - Program Renewal Well Underway

An eventful year! The healing Circle widened on several fronts.

'93 Happenings — As the year ended community outreach beyond Ka Ka Wis was widening and deepening. The community-services co-ordinator, and other Centre staff took part in Sharing Circle meetings with former and prospective clients in Ahousat, Opitsat and other communities. Outreach counsellors elsewhere on Vancouver Island were doing the same. In his spare time Dave Frank, night attendant at Ka Ka Wis, made follow-up calls to former clients, while intake-recorder Sherry Merk kept in touch with prospective client families.

- As requested by the Tla O Qui Aht First Nations' chief and council, elders and community workers, the Centre earmarked one fall session for client families living at Opitsat and Esowista (Long Beach). Speaking of local suicide attempts, alcohol and drug abuse, Chief Francis Frank challenged families: "It's time for you to start working on these issues, and begin working with the community.... Let's make it happen."

- A special newsletter was published for the dozen women clients and their children who came to the Single Moms' Summer Session. Clients contributed short comments, poems, art and the recipe for "Florence's Wonderful Doughnuts". Home addresses were listed so clients could keep in touch.

- Centre directors and staff decided to shorten the counselling program from six to four weeks on a trial basis. Shorter sessions would enable up to 72 client families to register yearly for counselling compared to the current average of 48. Families would spend less time away from homes, jobs and school. Waiting lists would shorten. These expected advantages persuaded Ka Ka Wis to take "a big step and a risk".

- An organizing committee was named to plan the Centre's 20th anniversary feast and celebration in early July 1994.

Comments Then & Later — "I would say it has served our people well," replied Nelson Keitlah, when the Co-chairman of the Central Region, Nuu-chah-nulth Tribal Council, was asked his opinion about the Ka Ka Wis program. He is the NTC representative for five coastal tribes — Ahousat, Hesquiat, Tla O Qui Aht (formerly called Clayoquot), Toquaht and Ucluelet.

"Ka Ka Wis has helped people get on the right track in wrestling with substance abuse in our homes," Mr. Keitlah stated. Unlike most other centres that treated individuals, Ka Ka Wis is "family oriented". He summed up: "Ka

Ka Wis is a catalyst, a very helpful and necessary catalyst in helping our people reach an honest recovery.... The Tribal Council supports Ka Ka Wis because of its good track record in dealing with our people."

- In the June issue of *TFN: "Living for a Better Tomorrow"* Delores Seitcher, alcohol-and-drug care worker, invited Tla O Qui Aht members to join Family Healing Circles: "As we are all aware, we have a lot of pain through suicides and death of our loved ones. A lot of our children hurt on some of the issues that have happened in our households.... This is an opportunity for us to work together. We can learn communication, budgeting, values and beliefs.... This is for anyone willing to learn different skills and values for personal growth."

- "I fully support the vision of Ka Ka Wis and the direction you're heading in terms of outreach treatment programming and after care," wrote Charlene Antinuk of the Valley Native Friendship Centre in Duncan. "I feel you're doing an excellent job of communicating with us and providing many openings for our input on services."

- "My goal is 80% sobriety and we're almost there," reported Edwin James, drug and alcohol counsellor working in Kyuquot, where the first family-healing plan for addicts took shape in the early 1970's. "We have a support group with 47 adults in it now. The only parties we have are sober parties. It is a miracle, considering how it was when I first came here."

1994 – Twenty Years of Healing: It's Time to Celebrate!

IV – What of the Future? Some Possibilities

By P.K.

In trying to envisage the future of Ka Ka Wis, I think it is important to look back to the past experiences and lessons of the Centre.

Over the years the program evolved and developed as it responded to the needs of the families and communities Ka Ka Wis serves. The initial idea to work with families has remained a constant. The idea of community development, which has resurfaced in the last three years, also was part of the original concept. The first proposal in 1973 was called the "Ka Ka Wis Family and Community Development Project". We now realize more than ever that community development is a must, and must remain a part of the Ka Ka Wis vision.

The Centre is a spiritual place. Many, if not all, of the staff over the years have seen spirituality as our core. The Christian element, AA spirituality, and native rituals and spirituality are coming together to form a broad base for the special spirituality of Ka Ka Wis. Spirituality is a person's reaching out to become the person one is meant to be. And that is what Ka Ka Wis is about.

Also, Ka Ka Wis has been a place of healing, of CHANGE, from the very beginning. Again, this is central to the Centre's reason for being.

With those four components — family, community, spirituality and healing — as givens, what Ka Ka Wis becomes is up to the creativity and good will of those associated with it in future years.

In the 1991 ADP assessment report, *Expanding the Ka Ka Wis Circle*, the Centre's future was envisioned as a gradual and respectful process of change from being an isolated, independent program to a project that promotes healing among workers and families **primarily** in their home communities. In the next 20 to 25 years, then, it is hoped that Ka Ka Wis will become a model community that performs various tasks to help people live full lives as healthy individuals, in healthy families, in healthy communities.

Healing Journeys

But what might this look like? Let's give our imaginations the freedom to dream some of the possibilities:

Families and individuals see their A&D counsellors (by now called "wellness workers") on a regular basis for two to six months, as they deal with their need to change some behaviour patterns. The wellness workers are in frequent contact with Ka Ka Wis for their own skills training, personal development and professional support. There is a partnership between Ka Ka Wis staff and these workers in local communities. Most families and individuals who are seeing wellness workers may overcome whatever is causing trouble in their lives, and need go no further. But for some others there may need to be special exercises or times (a weekend, a week, two weeks) to deal with specific problems or issues.

These families would have a growth plan (called a recovery plan today), and some time spent at Ka Ka Wis would be part of their overall plan. One problem, let us suppose, might be deep-seated grief over the loss of a family member. If we really want to let our imagination go, I could see that in 25 years one of our grief exercises might entail getting a person or family in touch with the deceased and being comforted through that meeting. Ka Ka Wis, after all, is a spiritual place.

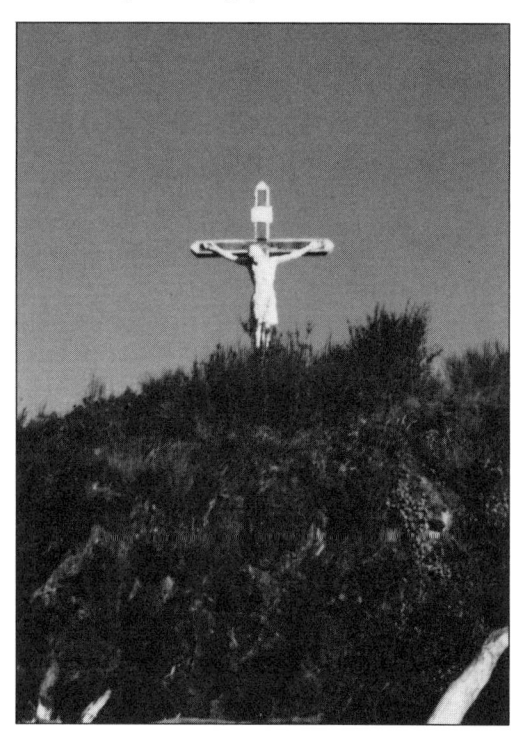

Another future activity might be a psychodrama about a community that was focused on prejudice or "female violence".

Whatever the issues may be 20 to 25 years from now, I hope Ka Ka Wis will be promoting wellness and growth — for all persons, families and their local communities.

Names and Numbers

Some Names Are Missing

Much effort was made to reach and talk with every living person who at some point helped the Ka Ka Wis story unfold in an important way. Most of those we reached responded willingly and warmly. A few did not return calls, and some we were unable to locate.

Why "Clients"?

A few advance readers of *Healing Journeys* questioned our use of the word "clients" in referring to native families who enrol for the Ka Ka Wis counselling program. "Find a more suitable word," these friendly critics suggested. Such as? "Customers"? "Patients"? "Guests"? These and other possible alternatives were considered and rejected as inappropriate. So the use of "clients" stays. Besides, after daily use for 20 years, the word has long since been accepted as suitable by aboriginal participants and Centre staff alike.

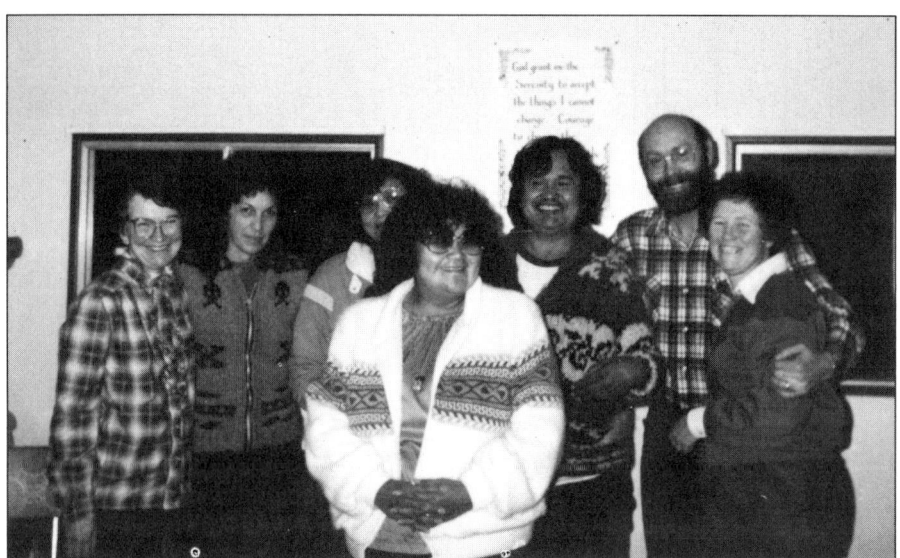

Left to Right: *Margaret Cantwell, Rose Head, Delores Seitcher, Mabel James, Ray Seitcher, Pat Koreski, Patricia Shreenan*

Members, Board of Directors

Unofficial Directors – December 1975 – July 1978

Stanley Douglas
Edwin Frank
Gertrude Frank
Gerry Guillet OMI
Darlene Haubrick
Roy Haiyupis
Dave Hawkes
Lorraine LaMarre SSA
Olivia Mae
Linda McConnel
Don McGinnis
Hugo Peterson
Geri Seinen

Official Directors – July 1978 – 1994

John Armstrong MD
Shamrock Atleo
Susan Atleo
Yvonne Bond
Gale Botting
Theresa Burkart
Rod Burke
Tom Cavanaugh OMI
Gary Celester
Eileen Charleson
Edgar Charlie
Tom Curley
Ben David
Dan David
Debbie David
Dave Dickson
Laurelle Doersam
Stanley Douglas
Mary Everson
Randy Fielder
John Fitzgerald OMI
Edwin Frank
Gertrude Frank
Louie Frank
Richard Foulkes MD
Grace George
Thomas George
Peter Greig
Gerry Guillet OMI
Beverly Hansen
Harvey Henderson MD
Jerry Jack Jr.
Louie Joseph
Wilma Keitlah
Pat Koreski
Joe Kranabetter
Roger Lacerte
Lise Larsen
Donald Lennox
Linus Lucas
Richard Lucas
Simon Lucas
Olivia Mae
Levi Martin
Moses Martin
Sharon Martin
Jim MacDonell OMI
Don McGinnis
Lydia Michael
Wayne Naka
Grace Neilsen
Margaret Rodgers
Jack Ryan OMI
Carol Sadler
Ruth Sadler
Wally Samuel
Geri Seinen
Millie Smith
Barbara Spencer
Lois Steven
Debbie Tom
Hugh Watts
Mark Webb
Debbie Williams

NOTE: Don McGinnis has been on the Board since it began and has served many terms as chairperson. Peter Greig has been a Board member for over 10 years. Our special thanks to both these dedicated members, and thanks also to all past and present directors.

Core Community, Centre Staff and Volunteers

JUNE 1971 Closure of the Old Christie Student Residence and staff departure

Core Community 1971 – 1975

Tom Cavanaugh OMI	Gerry Guillet OMI	Jim MacDonell OMI
Kathryn Erickson SSA	Lloyd and Francis Hooper	Lorraine LaMarre SSA
Joe Fligstein	Pat Koreski	Mary McGarrigle SSA
Louie, Eva Frank and family	Marjorie Kuntz CSJ	Alban and Rose Michael

Staff for Over Six Months 1976 – 1994

Judi Andrew	Archie Girvan	Sarah Peterson
Margaret Andrew	Kathy Girvan	Carol Proietti SSA
Wilfred Andrew	Elaine Greig/Killins	Marna Rogers SND
George Atleo	Gerry Guillet OMI	Jack Ryan OMI
Justine Ayre	Rose Head	Carol Sadler
Mervin Bannon	Harvey Henderson MD	Kathy Sawyer
Daryle Blackbird	Joe Hnasiewich	Delores Seitcher
Valerie Bob	Mabel James	Ray Seitcher
Debbie Burns	Marlene Joe	Patricia Shreenan SSA
Margaret Cantwell SSA	Ken Joe	Viola Sparvie
Bob Cato	Howard Johnston	Anita Tavera IHM
Maureen Cato	Lila Johnston	Derek Thompson
Tom Curley	Tom Johnston	Ellen Tolson
Mary David	Pat Koreski	Howard Tom Jr.
Tom David	Caroline Linitski	Joe Tom
Marie Donahue	J.C. Lucas	Martha Tom
Patricia Donovan SSA	Francis MacDonald OMI	Regina Tom
Gael Duchene	Jim MacDonell OMI	Rose Tom
Kathryn Erickson/Seitcher	Maxine Manson	Ginny Vandean/LeJeune
Dave Frank	Janis McDougall	Lynn Warner
Florence Frank	Harry McIntee	Ray Williams
Annie George	Sherry Merk	Sarah Williams
Lewis George	Reg O'Brien OMI	David Zryd

Staff Six Months or Less 1976 – 1994

George August	Delana George	Jerry Prazma OMI
J'Nette August	Grace George	Louie Sabbas Jr
Vern Bruhwiler	Jimmy Jack	Louie Sabbas Sr
Ike Campbell	Murray John Jr	Carol Savage
Lisa Charleson	Betty Keitlah	Martin Saxey
Kathleen Daly	Annie Loutit	Dean Sevold
Cecil Dawson	Mike Marshall	Sandra Seymour
Richard Donahue	Pat McClary	Carol Tom
Annette Favelle	Jane McDiarmid	Anna Vance
Catherine (Ginger) Frank	Randy McKay	Martin Vance
Elmer Frank	Ben Peters	Loretta Williams
Louie Frank	Jack Peterson	Francis Zeni
Wilfred Frank	Jeannine Pineau	

Over the years between 1983 - 1993, more than 50 different people not listed here worked on CEIC grants, UIC enhancement grants or summer youth grants. Many of the physical improvements to the facilities were made possible through these dedicated workers. As well, new friends were made and fun times had. Our thanks to all these unnamed workers.

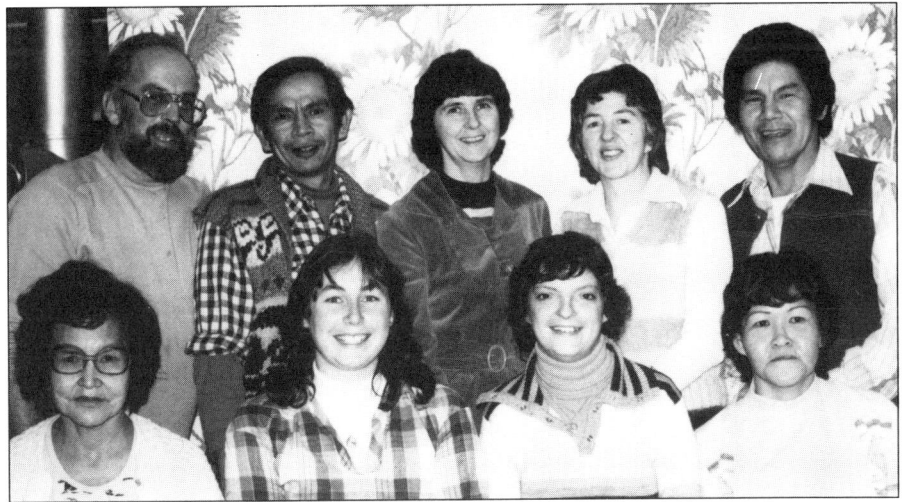

Front row: *Sarah Williams, Janis McDougall, Debbie Burns, Margaret Andrew.*
Back row: *Gerry Guillet, Ray Williams, Patricia Donovan, Lorraine LaMarre, Wilfred Andrew, Sr.*

Left to Right:
Tom Cavanaugh,
Frances Hooper,
Lloyd Hooper,
Ruth Little,
Marjorie Kuntz,
Kathy Erickson,
Mary McGarrigle,
Gerry Guillet,
a visiting couple,
Jim MacDonell

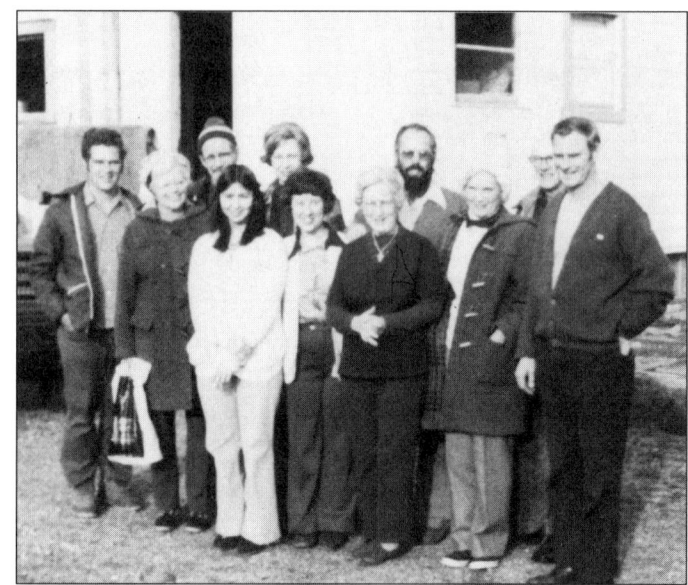

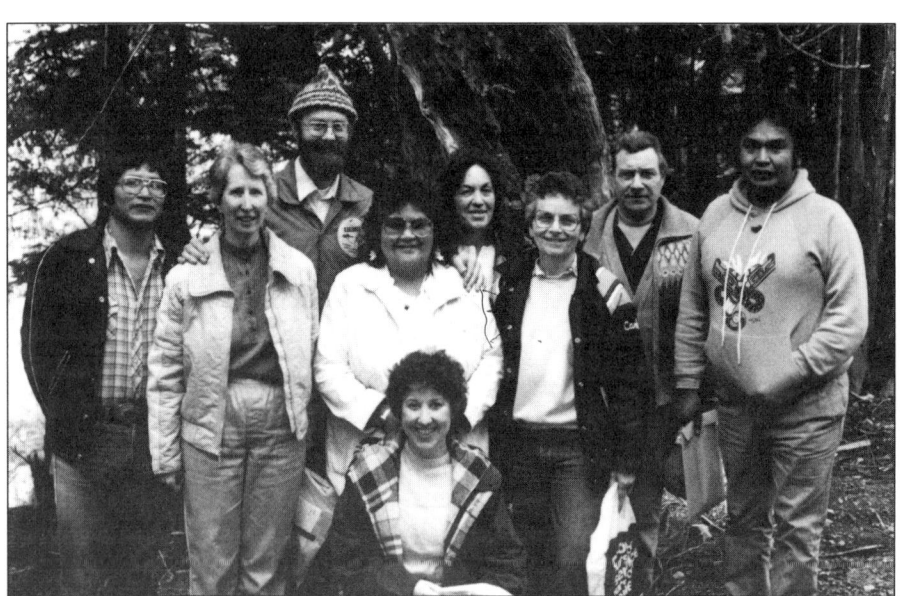

Left to Right: Tom David, Marna Rogers, Pat Koreski, Mabel James, Kathy Erickson (seated), Rose Head, Carol Proietti, Jacky Ryan, Ray Seitcher.

Sample Program Exercise

Torn Spirits

Purpose: To help clients recognize (using a visual demonstration) that unkind words "tear one's spirit" and that kind words can "help rebuild it."

Material: A small piece of paper for each person (4 X 6 in. approximately), one large piece of construction paper (12 X 18 in.), tape.

Time: Approximately one hour.

Part One: The leader instructs everyone:

Look at the scraps of paper - all are different. Some look like garbage. Look at the big piece - smooth, untorn, like the spirit of a new-born baby. When someone says or does something to the baby, it is like a little of their spirit is torn off and dies (like when an older child shows jealousy, when they are hit, when they are yelled at). Tear off a large piece and let it fall to the ground. What other things "tear your spirit"? Invite everyone in the circle to take a turn saying something which they heard or said to someone which "tore their spirit." As things are said, each person tears their papers, and the leader tears from the large piece.

Draw attention to how small the papers are getting.

Part Two: "Build the spirit." Ask, "Can we undo the damage? How?" (ie., saying or doing nice things, etc.) As each suggestion is made, invite the person making it to pick up one of the pieces of the large paper and tape it back onto a small piece which has been taped onto the board. The taped tears are the scars and marks which are always with us, but the spirit can be built up again.

Discussion: In the whole circle, ask for comments and discussion.

KA KA WIS FOUNDATION FUND

The operation of the Ka ka Wis Family Development Centre is presently funded almost entirely by government grants. In order to ensure our future and some independence, Ka Ka Wis would like to set up a Foundation Fund within the Vancouver Foundation. Revenues from this Fund would help support Centre programs. Income-tax receipts for your contribution would be provided. If you would like to donate to this fund and/or help with fund-raising, please complete the following form and send it to :

Executive Director,
Ka Ka Wis Family Development Centre,
Box 17, TOFINO, B.C.
V0R 2Z0

Yes, I would like to donate $____ to the Ka Ka Wis Foundation Fund.

☐ My cheque is enclosed.   ☐ Perhaps at a later date.

☐ I would like to run or support fund-raising activities in my community.

☐ I would like to set aside a portion of my estate for this fund.

Name(s) _____

Address _____

Postal Code _____

Telephone (___) _____

Fax _____